Gaa-izhi-miinigoowizid a'aw Anishinaabe

What We Were Given as Anishinaabe

GAA-IZHI-MIINIGOOWIZID A'AW ANISHINAABE
What We Were Given as Anishinaabe

Lee *Obizaan* Staples
As told to Chato *Ombishkebines* Gonzalez

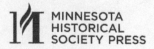
MINNESOTA
HISTORICAL
SOCIETY PRESS

mnhspress.org

The Minnesota Historical Society Press is a member of the Association of University Presses.

Manufactured in the United States of America

10 9 8 7 6 5 4 3 2 1

♾ The paper used in this publication meets the minimum requirements of the American National Standard for Information Sciences—Permanence for Printed Library Materials, ANSI Z39.48-1984.

International Standard Book Number
ISBN: 978-1-68134-267-2 (paper)

Library of Congress Control Number: 2023935077

CONTENTS

Gaa-izhi-miinigoowizid a'aw Anishinaabe

What We Were Given as Anishinaabe

INTRODUCTION

For some Anishinaabe families living in what is now considered the Southwestern Ojibwe territory of Minnesota, Wisconsin, and parts of Michigan and Ontario, two generations or more have passed since children grew up with the teachings and ceremonies described in this collection. As Chi-Obizaan Maakawaadizid, Lee Staples, knows all too well, the behavior and the demeanor of our children is often a reflection of the teachings they receive in their homes. He encourages the parent generation to bring their children to Anishinaabe ceremonies and to teach them about the Anishinaabe spiritual way of life. Obizaan reminds us that our children will do what we do, and it is important to remember to show them the beauty of the life we have been given as Anishinaabe.

Through our catastrophic and traumatizing experience with colonization and external cultural forces, many of our families and communities have lost touch with the ceremonies and teachings put in place to empower our children and establish a relationship with the *Manidoog*—and with the spiritually based thinking behind them. We have heard certain things growing up, like "Don't whistle at night!" or "Make sure you have holes in your baby's moccasins!" though we may never have been told the reasoning behind such cultural teachings. In this collection, Obizaan describes the teachings and various ceremonies—from pre-birth through the coming of age—that we were given as Anishinaabe for our children. He oftentimes explains the spiritual as well as the practical reasons for why they are the way they are.

As someone who has been fortunate enough to listen to Obizaan reiterate these teachings time and again, I have had the pleasure of hearing him remind many of our relatives of the importance of our spiritually based mindset as a people. We have heard his renditions of the *waabooz* in a gunnysack, kicking and screaming to get out, and the comparison he makes to the Anishinaabe spirit that isn't nurtured. He encourages us to attend ceremonies and learn to speak our language, as those are both key to properly nurturing our Anishinaabe spirits within us.

Obizaan uses the phrase *spiritual bankruptcy* to describe our Anishinaabe people having no spiritual basis in their lives and struggling to find peace and satisfaction in daily life. Many times, this spiritual bankruptcy leads our relatives to turn to other forms of satisfaction, oftentimes overusing alcohol and other mind-altering substances. Other times, our relatives carry their grief and the pain they have experienced through loss without a proper channel to relieve it. When it is not dealt with in the proper manner, this pain and suffering can come out sideways and hurt the ones we love the most. As social and health problems like addiction, child welfare, domestic violence, and diabetes continue to mount for Anishinaabe people and their communities, the general tribal response is to write a grant and create a program to combat the current crisis. But these efforts often fall short, since they do not properly deal with the root of the problems. If we reflect on the current shape and health of our modern Anishinaabe communities from a spiritually based Anishinaabe perspective, it seems obvious that many of our problems are the direct result of not knowing or following our traditional teachings.

Obizaan reminds us to begin our teachings with our children when they are small, although it is never too late. The sooner we foster a relationship with the *Manidoog*, the better chance we have at finding the path that was intended for each of us individually and the less suffering we experience. One of Obizaan's greatest fears is seeing the day when Anishinaabe children have no regard for their ceremonies and teachings, no regard for their elders, and no regard for their fellow Anishinaabe. Sadly, this day has already arrived for some families in some communities. Our traditional ways are endangered, and individuals like Obizaan who hold on to these teachings are becoming fewer with the passing of each generation. This reality makes the importance of these teachings and the publication of this book that much more urgent.

The chapters that appear here are a collection of articles, some previously published in tribal newspapers in the Southwestern Ojibwe region. Many of the drafts have served as curriculum for our Ojibwe-language immersion classrooms, tribal language and culture programs, and college-level language and culture classes. They appear here in a fresh, convenient bilingual format, compiled in chronological order and followed by a glossary. Obizaan and Ombishkebines (his assistant, Chato Gonzalez) have scoured these pages, and I served as a reviewer and spellchecker for many of the original newspaper articles as well as this recent compilation.

As some of the premier published Ojibwe authors, Obizaan and Ombishkebines have developed many of their own conventions with regard to the written representation of Ojibwemowin, based solely on Obizaan's preferences for how certain things appear in print. For example, Obizaan prefers to capitalize certain words like *Manidoo* (spirit) that are capitalized in the Ojibwe text, and others like *Winter Legends* are capitalized in the English text. Other terms, like *chi-mookomaan* (white man) are not capitalized in either language, following Obizaan's preference. He reminds us regularly that we can define our own parameters as a people, especially with regard to our language, and we should refrain from the common tendency to put our colonizer, the *chi-mookomaan*, on a pedestal. Choosing *not* to capitalize such words is one example of how Obizaan defies such tendencies.

Language learners and enthusiasts will be delighted by this book's contents, as Obizaan is renowned for his intricate and sophisticated vocabulary and his eloquent descriptions, both signatures of our most distinguished speakers. Readers should also keep in mind that the translations given by Obizaan here are largely free, running translations, which might differ from the literal thinking of learners. On page 34–35, *mindimooyenyiban nebowa ogii-gikendaanan mashkikiwan imaa wendinigaadenig imaa bagwaj* is translated as *that old lady knew medicines that **you** could pick from the wild*. Readers should be aware that the "you" is implied in the Ojibwe and isn't literal. Such supplementation in the English is often necessary, as literal renderings would be clumsy. Consider the following (p. 62–63):

> *Gomaapii dash waabamind iniw asemaan da-miinaa.*
> When the parents see them at a later date, they can give that person some tobacco.

The sentence is rooted in a context, specifically the context of protocol followed for an absent namesake at a naming ceremony. Nowhere in the sentence is a word for *parents*. The literal translation, *Later on when s/he is seen, they will give h/ tobacco*, is vague and doesn't quite capture the full meaning expressed. Despite Obizaan's knack for providing illustrative translations, he reminds us that "the English language is inadequate for translating Ojibwemowin."

Advanced learners of Ojibwemowin will notice variation at the vocabulary level, as Obizaan's preferred terms appear instead of the perhaps more common forms. Words like *maamandoogwaason* (a quilt), *waazakonenjiganaaboo* (gasoline), *obiizikaaganiwaan* (their clothes), and others are Obizaan's preferred ways of saying the more standard forms of *maawandoogwaason, waasamoo-bimide,* and *obiizikiiganiwaan*. Also noticeable in the text is Obizaan's natural variation with personal prefixes, going back and forth between *ingii-* and *nigii-, nimb-* and *nib-, ind-,* and *nind-* with no real pattern of their distribution. Language learners who have been taught to focus on these subtleties may be surprised to see such variation exists among individuals.

Other notable language-specific points of discussion have been observed in Obizaan's other books, including the marking of dependent noun stems, such as *niwiiji-anishinaabe/niij-anishinaabe*. Certain things about Obizaan's speech are best appreciated by hearing, rather than reading, such as his tendency to doubly mark the plural

with inanimate intransitive verbs like *agoojigaade**wanoon,*** which
has a sort of fancy ring to it when Obizaan says it. Certain English
translations given here reflect Obizaan's English, like the absence
of a location with the verb *put* (It is not necessary to put a bowl or
maybe bowls for the close relatives, p. 26–27). Readers from more
northern Ojibwe backgrounds may notice certain Southwestern
Ojibwe–specific uses of verbs like *wiiji'* (vta, play with h/), differ-
ing from its use in the north of *help h/,* or with verbs pertaining
to the mouth (=doon/=doone), which are used by Obizaan and
others in the more southern regions with no final vowel =e: *Gego
aabidaanagidoongen naa gego onzaamidoongen* (Do not talk too much
or be mouthy, p. 128–29).

Advanced language learners will love and marvel at the mor-
phological complexity of the participles Obizaan and others
from his region are famous for. Where second-language learners
struggle with spontaneous mastery of structural aspects of the
grammar such as participant arrangement and verbal direction, or proximate/obviative shifts across a narrative, Obizaan
delivers significant lessons that transcend simple language
teaching. Insisting on always teaching his students meaningful,
Anishinaabe-minded, spiritually based substance, Obizaan has
given his readers and his students to come an awesome collection
of teachings on both the spiritual way of the Anishinaabe and the
intricate language he uses to teach it.

Before he became an elder, I doubt Obizaan ever imagined he
would one day have to compile all of these teachings into a book.
The practices were simply too well known. But culture change and
language shift have both happened within his lifetime. While it
may be easy to dwell on loss and sulk in misery, many of us choose
to celebrate the amount of traditional Anishinaabe knowledge we
have managed to maintain in spite of our experience and the inten-
tional effort to rob us and cheat us out of our way of life. Thanks
to knowledge keepers like Obizaan, future generations of Anishinaabe have access to this older, perhaps better way of being, better

way of seeing the world, and better understanding of our cultural and spiritual identity.

Chi-wawiingezi a'aw Chi-obizaan ina'oonaad Anishinaaben niigaan minik omaa wezhibii'igaadeg yo'ow mazina'iganing. Geget igo gizhawenimigonaan a'aw akiwenzii.

Michael *Migizi* Sullivan Sr., PhD
6zd Onaabani-giizis 2023
Odaawaa-zaaga'iganing

1 I'IW AKEYAA GE-IZHI-MINWAABADAK OMAA WEZHIBII'IGAADEG

[1] Mii omaa mazina'iganing ani-dazhindamaan anooj
a'aw Anishinaabe gaa-miinigoowizid ge-ondinigenid inow
oniijaanisan miinawaa awegwen igo weshki-bimaadizinijin
da-ni-naadamaagoowizinid anooj akeyaa ani-biindaakoojigenid.
Gaawiin gaye nimichi-giizhitoosiin omaa ani-dazhindamaan.
Ishke a'aw akiwenziiyiban, indedeyiban, Ogimaawab, gii-
izhinikaazo. Ingii-pabaa-wiijiiwaa gii-nandomind da-ni-
ganoodamawaad iniw Anishinaaben ani-asemaakenid.

[2] Ishke dash mii imaa wenji-gikendamaan o'ow gaagiigidowin
gaa-achigaadeg. Ishke ishkweyaang gii-onjikaamagadini gii-
gikinoo'amawind a'aw akiwenziiyiban, mii dash imaa aazhita
gii-gikinoo'amawid gaye niin. Ishke bezhig a'aw nizigosiban,
Nechii'awaasong, nebowa ogii-gikendaan anooj akeyaa ani-izhi-
gaagiigidong ani-asemaakenid inow Anishinaaben. Mii gaye a'aw
mindimooyenyiban nebowa gaa-gikinoo'amawid.

[3] Ishke dash a'aw Anishinaabe ge-ni-izhichigepan, mii
iwidi endanakamigizid a'aw Anishinaabe ani-asemaaked,
mii iwidi ge-izhiwinaapan inow oniijaanisan. Ishke mii i'iw
gaa-toodaagooyaan niin. Mii imaa gaa-taniziyaan gii-pabaa-
wiijiiwagwaa ingiw gaa-nitaawigi'ijig gii-naazikaagewaad
endazhi-niimi'idiiked a'aw Anishinaabe. Mii-go gaye iwidi
Aazhoomog, gii-ozhigewaad i'iw wiigiwaam gii-ozhitoowaad
da-ayaayaang imaa megwaa gii-midewiwaad.

[4] Ishke gaye a'aw abinoojiinh, asemaan naa wiisiniwin
atamawind, mii gaye gaa-toodaagooyaan. Ingii-
wiiyawen'enyikaagoo biinish gaye gii-sagaswe'idiwaad
apii gii-oshki-nitooyaan gegoo. Miinawaa mii eta-go gii-
ojibwemotaagooyaan gaa-tazhi-ganawenimigooyaan.

1 HOW THIS WRITTEN MATERIAL CAN BE PUT TO GOOD USE

[1] In this book, I am talking about the various ceremonies that are given to the Anishinaabe to help their children and other youth in which their tobacco is offered up. I am not just creating what I am saying. I traveled with the old man, my late father, John Benjamin, when he was asked to speak for the Anishinaabe's tobacco.

[2] That is why I know the talk that goes with these ceremonies. What the old man was taught came from the past, and then he in turn taught me what he was given. Also one of my late aunts, Mary Churchill-Benjamin, knew a lot of the talk that went with various offerings that the Anishinaabe made. It was this old lady that taught me a lot, also.

[3] What the Anishinaabe people should do is take their children to the various ceremonies that we have been given. That is what was done to me. I traveled with those old people as they attended the various ceremonial dances. They also built a wigwam in *Aazhoomog*, where we stayed while they partook in the *midewiwin* lodge.

[4] Tobacco and food is offered up to help a child, and that was what was done for me. They gave me my namesakes and had a feast for my first kill. They also only spoke Ojibwe in the home that I was raised in.

[5] A'aw mindimooyenyiban, nimaamaayiban, mii i'iw
gaa-izhichiged gabe-biboon gii-aadizookawid. Ishke gaye
ingii-waabandaan gaa-izhi-apiitendamowaad Anishinaabe
gaa-miinigoowizid. Mii-go apane a'aw mindimooyenyiban
gii-ozhitood iniw maamandoogwaasonan naa-go gaye iniw
manidoominensikaan waa-pagijigewaad. Ishke dash mii imaa
gii-waabandamaan gaa-ina'oonwewizid a'aw Anishinaabe
ge-ni-apenimod.

[6] Ishke dash imaa maa minik igo nigii-ni-nishwanaajiwebinige
bimiwidooyaan i'iw nibimaadiziwin gii-ni-aabajitooyaan i'iw
minikwewin nebowa a'aw Anishinaabe eni-nishwanaaji'igod.
Azhigwa gaa-moonendamaan da-ni-boonitooyaan wenda-
inigaa'igoyaan, mii imaa gii-gikendamaan ge-apa'iweyaan
da-ni-naadamaagoowiziyaan. Ishke dash mii imaa gii-ni-
mikwendamaan inigokwekamig gaa-waabandamaan a'aw
Anishinaabe gaa-miinigoowizid miinawaa ge-ni-apenimod.
Mii dash imaa gaa-apa'iweyaan agana dash noongom
wenji-izhiwebiziyaan.

[7] Ishke dash ani-dazhindamaan o'ow mii imaa ani-
ayaangwaamimag a'aw niwiiji-anishinaabe da-ni-waabanda'aad
inow oniijaanisan i'iw akeyaa gaa-izhi-ina'oonwewiziyang
da-babaa-izhiwinaad aaniindi-go ani-asemaaked a'aw
Anishinaabe. Ishke dash eni-gichi-aya'aawinid oniijaanisan,
giishpin ani-nishwanaajiwebinigenid ani-bimiwidoonid
obimaadiziwin, mii imaa gaye wiin da-ni-gikendang da-ni-
apa'iwed da-ni-naadamaagoowizid.

[5] The old lady, my late mother, what she did was tell me the Winter Legends throughout the winter. I also saw the respect for what we were given as Anishinaabe. That old lady was constantly sewing quilts and doing beadwork, which was their offering at the various ceremonies that they went to. It was there that I saw the teachings that were given to the Anishinaabe to rely on.

[6] There was a period there where I messed up in my life by using alcohol, which has been a downfall to the Anishinaabe. When I began to realize that I needed to leave the alcohol alone, I knew where to run to for help. It is then that I remembered all that the Anishinaabe had been given to rely on. I ran to all of that for help, which is why today I am halfway sane.

[7] As I talk about this, I am strongly encouraging the Anishinaabe to show their children what we have been given as Anishinaabe and take them to ceremonies. As the children get older, and if their children have problems in their future not carrying their life in a good way, they will also know where to run for help.

[8] Ishke dash gaye ani-nitaawigi'ind a'aw abinoojiinh o'ow akeyaa, oga-wenda-gikendaan anishinaabewid ayaang imaa dibendaagozid ani-gaagiiwozhitoosig i'iw bimaadizid. Ishke noongom nebowa a'aw Anishinaabe-abinoojiinh ani-izhiwebizid dibishkoo-go ani-gaagiiwozhitoo. Gaawiin dibishkoo ogikendanziin i'iw dedebinawe gaa-ina'oonwewizid anishinaabewid.

[9] Booch a'aw bemaadizid da-ayaang dibendaagozid. Ishke dash mii i'iw nebowa a'aw weshki-bimaadizid wenji-odaapinang babaa-wiiji'iwed *gangs* ezhi-wiinjigaadegin. Ishke dash wiin a'aw weshki-bimaadizid weweni gaa-nitaawigi'ind gii-gikinoo'amawind gaa-izhi-miinigoowiziyang anishinaabewiyang, mii i'iw wiin wenda-gikendang omaa dibendaagozid anishinaabeng akeyaa.

[8] If a child is raised in this manner, he will definitely know that he is Anishinaabe and not wander in life as if he is lost. What is happening nowadays is a lot of our Anishinaabe youth are wandering about in life as if they are lost and not connecting anywhere. They are not aware of what we were truly given as Anishinaabe.

[9] All people must have a place where they belong. It is why a lot of our Anishinaabe young people today adopt the gang lifestyle as it is called. But our young people who have been brought up in the old way and who were taught our ways, they know that they belong with the Anishinaabe and are a part of that life.

2 DABWAA-ONDAADIZID

[1] Dabwaa-ondaadizid a'aw Anishinaabe, mii omaa apii giizhaa wii-ni-dazhindamaan i'iw bimaadiziwin. Geget gii-chi-ina'oonwewizi gii-miinigoowizid i'iw bimaadiziwin a'aw Anishinaabe.

[2] Ishke aabiding ingezikwendaan owapii gii-wiij'ayaawag a'aw mindimooyenyiban, nizigosiban. Namanj gaa-izhiwebiziwaanen gaa-izhi-wiindamawag a'aw mindimooyenyiban, "Geget nindinigaaz", nigii-inaa. Mii i'iw gaa-izhi-naniibikimid, "Gaawiin gidinigaazisiin. Gibimaadiziwin gidayaan," nigii-ig.

[3] Mii inow Manidoon ena'oonigojin a'aw Anishinaabe i'iw bimaadiziwin, mii iwidi wenjikaamagadinig. Mii dash i'iw weweni ge-onji-ganawendang obimaadiziwin a'aw Anishinaabe da-ni-minochiged megwaa imaa bibizhaagiid omaa akiing. Gakina a'aw bemaadizid odayaawaan inow Manidoon zhewenimigojin, genawenimigojin igaye megwaa omaa ayaad omaa akiing. Mii ow gaa-onji-wiindamaagoowiziyang weweni da-ni-doodawang a'aw giwiiji-bimaadiziiminaan. Giishpin maazhi-doodawang giwiiji-bimaadiziiminaan, mii inow Manidoon mayaazhi-doodawimangin mii inow Manidoon zhewenimigojin, miinawaa gaa-miinigojin i'iw bimaadiziwin.

2 BEFORE BIRTH

[1] It is here ahead of time I want to talk about life before an Anishinaabe person is born. It was a great gift when Anishinaabe were given life.

[2] I recall this one time when I lived with that old lady, my late aunt. I do not know what happened to me when I told that old lady, "I am really pitiful," I said to her. And then she scolded me. "You are not pitiful. You have your life," she said to me.

[3] The spirits give the Anishinaabe life; that is where our lives come from. That is why Anishinaabe should take care of their life and live well while they are here on earth. Everyone living has spirits that watch over them and take care of them while they are here on earth. That is why we are told to respect our fellow human beings. If we treat our fellow human beings with disrespect, we are disrespecting those spirits that have compassion for them and also the ones that gave them life.

[4] Anishinaabewi a'aw biinjina eyaawang a'aw gijichaagwanaan.
Mii ingiw Manidoog gaa-inaakonigejig i'iw akeyaa Anishinaabeng
da-ni-izhi-bimaadiziyang. Ishke ingiw Manidoog geget
ogii-shawenimaawaan inow odanishinaabemiwaan gii-
miinigoowiziyang ge-ni-inweyang da-ojibwemoyang, naa gaye
gii-miinigoowiziyang i'iw akeyaa ge-ni-izhichigeyang ani-
biindaakoojigeyang miinawaa i'iw ge-izhi-bimiwidooyang i'iw
bimaadiziyang. Mii iw ge-ni-ayaangwaamitooyangiban miinawaa
ge-ni-apiitendamangiban. Gigii-miinigonaanig ingiw Manidoog
i'iw akeyaa ge-izhi-bimaadiziyang. Mii i'iw ge-minokaagoyang
imaa biinjina gijichaagwanaaning.

[5] Gaawiin gidaa-aanawendanziimin ingiw Manidoog gaa-
izhi-ina'oonaawaad inow odanishinaabemiwaan. Gaawiin
gidaa-debwetawaasiwaanaan a'aw wayaabishkiiwed. Geget
aanoodizi wii-wayezhimaad inow Anishinaaben. Gaawiin gidaa-
mamoosiimin a'aw wayaabishkiiwed ezhitwaad.

[6] Gigii-miinigonaanig ingiw Manidoog ge-izhitwaayang
anishinaabewiyang. Ishke mamooyang i'iw wayaabishkiiwed
ezhitwaad, gaawiin imaa biinjina gijichaagwanaaning
zakab giga-izhi-ayaasiimin. Gidaa-migwanaadizimin imaa
biinjina. Mii o'ow apane gaa-izhi-gikinoo'amawiwaad gaa-
nitaawigi'ijig. Gii-ikidowag, "Ani-mamood a'aw Anishinaabe
i'iw akeyaa ezhitwaanid inow wayaabishkiiwen, gaawiin
da-izhaasiin iwidi eni-izhaanid inow gidinawemaaganinaanin
gaagwiinawaabaminaagozinid omaa akiing."

[7] Ishke i'iw maajaa'iweyaan, moozhag nibi-noondaan a'aw
Anishinaabe i'iw bakaan izhi-maajaa'ind, gaawiin izhaasiin
iwidi gidinawemaaganinaanin ezhaanid gegoo izhiwebizinid.
Mii-go omaa izhi-waabanjigaazonid inow ojichaagwan omaa
endaad a'aw bakaan gaa-izhi-maajaa'ind. Gaawiin ingoji
izhaasiiwan inow ojichaagwan.

[4] That spirit we have within us is Anishinaabe. It was the spirits that made the decision that we should live an Anishinaabe life. The spirits really had a lot of compassion for their Anishinaabe when they gave us a way to sound, to speak the Ojibwe language, and also we were given a specific way to offer our tobacco and live our lives. It is that life that we should take special care of and think highly of. It was the spirits that gave us the way to live our lives. That is what will make our spirit inside of us feel really good.

[5] We should not view what Anishinaabe were given by the spirits to be inadequate. We should not believe what the white man says as being the truth. They have a strong desire to deceive the Anishinaabe. We should not take the white man's way of life.

[6] The spirits gave us our own way of life as Anishinaabe. If we were to take the white man's way of life, the spirit inside of us would not be at peace. We would be unsettled within. This is what my parents always taught me. They said, "If an Anishinaabe takes the white man's way of life, he will not go where our relatives go when they are no longer seen on earth."

[7] When I do a funeral, I often hear that Anishinaabe who are sent off a different way do not go where our relatives go when something happens to them. Their spirit is seen in their home after they have been sent off a different way. Their spirit does not go anywhere.

[8] A'aw mindimooyenyiban, gaa-nitaawigi'id, mii i'iw gaa-izhichiged azhigwa besho enendaagwadinig inow ikwewan wii-ayaawaad inow oniijaanisan, mii imaa gii-naadamaaged a'aw mindimooyenyiban. Nimikwendaan mii eta-go a'aw akiwenziiyiban naa gaye niin imaa gii-ayaayaang niibaa-dibik imaa endaayaang, gaawiin a'aw mindimooyenyiban gii-ayaasiin.

[9] Mii iwidi gii-paa-naadamawaad inow ikwewan oniijaanisan waa-ayaawaajin. Mii dash a'aw mindimooyenyiban gaa-izhi-gikinoo'amawaad inow ikwewan gegishkawaanijin oniijaanisiwaan. Ogii-kagaanzomaan inow ikwewan moozhag da-mamaajiinid da-anokiinid imaa ayaanid. Gego da-wii-bizaanishinziiwag ingiw ikwewag. Anooj igo omaa da-anokiiwaad imaa ayaawaad. Giishpin apane bizaanishing a'aw ikwe megwaa bimiwinaad inow oniijaanisan, da-gagwaadagitoo azhigwa iwapii ayaawaad inow oniijaanisan. Miinawaa nizigosiban ogii-izhi-gikinoo'amawaan inow ikwewan, "Azhigwa ayaawad a'aw giniijaanis, gego aazhikweken, gaawiin gigii-aazhikwesiin iwapii gii-ozhi'eg giniijaanisiwaa."

[10] Nigii-pi-noodaan igaye aanind ingiw ikwewag ogii-nagamotawaawaan inow oniijaanisiwaan megwaa imaa biinjina gii-pimiwinaawaad.

[11] Miinawaa gaye imaa maajaa'iweng, mii imaa gii-gikina'amawindwaa, gaawiin odaa-bi-waabamaasiwaawaan gaa-ishkwaa-ayaanijin. Gegoo daa-izhiwebiziwan inow abinoojiinyan bemiwinaawaajin.

[12] Ayaapii iko gaye ingiw ikwewag gegishkawaajig inow oniijaanisiwaan ninandomigoog da-gaagiigidotamawagwaa inow asemaan miinawaa wiisiniwin ininamawaawaad inow Manidoon weweni da-naadamaagoowiziwaad weweni da-bi-dagoshininid oniijaanisiwaan.

[8] The old lady who raised me helped the women who were about to deliver their babies. I remember that it was only that old man and I who were home at night, and that old lady was not there.

[9] The old lady would be out helping the women who were about to give birth. She would also teach the women who were pregnant. She would encourage these women to move often and to work during their pregnancy. The women should not lie around. They should work on different things while they are pregnant. If a woman is always lying around while she is pregnant, she will have a difficult time during her delivery. My aunt would also teach the women, "When you are delivering your baby, you should not scream; because you did not scream when you and your old man were making your baby."

[10] I also heard that some women sing to their babies while they are pregnant.

[11] And also at the funerals, the women that were pregnant were warned not to view the deceased. They were told if they did, something could happen to the baby that they are carrying.

[12] Sometimes pregnant women will ask me to talk for their tobacco and food that they are offering to the spirits to help them and for their baby to arrive safely.

[13] Miinawaa gaye nigezikwendaan gii-wiindamaagoowiziyaan; gego gidaa-wii-panaajitoosiinan ingiw bineshiinyag owadiswaniwaan miinawaa inow owaawanoomiwaan. Ingii-igoo "Ishke ingoding abinoojiinyag gaye giin gidaa-ni-ayaawaag, mii imaa da-bi-azheshkaagoyamban."

[13] I also recall when I was told not to destroy the bird's nests or their eggs. I was told, "Someday you too could have babies; and it is at that time it could come back on you."

3 WANI'IND ABINOOJIINYENS

[1] Azhigwa a'aw ikwe wani'aad inow oniijaanisensan
bemiwinaajin, odaa-ni-naniizaanenimaan inow Chi-
mookomaani-mashkikiiwininiwan. Ishke gaawiin a'aw
wayaabishkiiwed gegoo odapiitendanziin i'iw akeyaa gaa-izhi-
gikinoo'amaagoowiziyang anishinaabewiyang.

[2] Mii i'iwapii gaa-ozhi'ind a'aw abinoojiinyens, mii-go
omaa gii-ayaanid inow ojichaagwan. Daa-gagwedwe a'aw
ikwe da-giiwewinaad inow abinoojiinyensan gaa-wani'aajin
megwaa gii-pimiwinaapan. Ishke gaawiin gikendaagwasinini
ge-doodawindwaabanen inow abinoojiinyensan weni'aawaajin
ingiw ikwewag megwaa bimiwinaawaad. Maagizhaa gaye ingiw
Chi-mookomaani-mashkikiiwininiwag epaginaawaagwen
inow abinoojiinyensan iwidi endazhi-apagiji-ziigwebinigeng.
Maagizhaa gaye anooj odoodawaawaadogenan inow
abinoojiinyensan giishkizhwaawaad, aana-wii-ondinamowaad
nawaj wii-gagwe-gikendamowaad gegoo.

[3] Booch da-maajaa'ind a'aw abinoojiinyens, giishpin
maajaa'aasiwind a'aw abinoojiinyens, mii-go omaa da-baa-
gaagiiwozhitoonid inow ojichaagwan omaa akiing.

3 THE DEATH OF A CHILD

[1] When a woman loses her baby while she is pregnant, she should be wary of the white doctors. The white man does not have respect for our teachings and what we were given as Anishinaabe.

[2] At the time of conception the baby has a spirit. The woman should ask to take home the fetus of the baby that she has lost. Who knows what might be done to these babies that these women have lost and miscarried. Maybe the white man will just throw the baby in the garbage, or maybe they are doing research, cutting the baby up to learn something new.

[3] It is necessary to send off the spirit of the baby; if the spirit is not sent off, his spirit will be wandering with no place to go here on earth.

[4] Mii dash omaa apii wii-ni-dazhindamaan i'iw gaagiigidowin gaa-achigaadeg ani-maajaa'ind a'aw abinoojiinyens gaa-wani'aajin a'aw ikwe megwaa gigishkawaad. Ishke gaa-ikidowaad ingiw akiwenziiyibaneg, mii iw izhi-gwayak iwidi wenji-izhaad a'aw abinoojiinyens iwidi ezhaawaad gidinawemaaganinaanig gegoo izhiwebiziwaad miinawaa wenji-noogitaasig omaa akiing, ogii-misawaabamigoon inow Manidoon gaa-onji-inendaagozid izhi-gwayak da-izhaad iwidi a'aw abinoojiinyens. Azhigwa ani-dagoshimoonod iwidi, mii inow Manidoon da-ina'oonigod a'aw abinoojiinyens gegoo gaa-onji-inendaagozid izhi-gwayak da-ni-izhaad iwidi gidinawemaaganinaanig eyaawaad, Gaagige-minawaanigoziwining ezhi-wiinjigaadeg.

[5] Ishke gaawiin gegoo ogii-wanendanziinaawaa ingiw Manidoog. Mii-go gii-atoowaad ge-ni-naadamaagod a'aw abinoojiinyens iwidi izhi-gwayak gii-inendaagozid da-ni-izhaad. Ishke a'aw Manidoo iwidi genawenimaad gidinawemaaganinaanin iwidi eyaanijin odayaawaan inow Manidoon nayaadamaagojin miinawaa genawenimaad inow abinoojiinyensan. Mii dash a'aw Gaagige-oshkiniigikwe. Mii a'aw ba-izhinizha'igaazod omaa, mii dash a'aw eni-dakonaajin inow abinoojiinyensan weweni da-dagoshimoono'aad iwidi eyaawaad gidinawemaaganinaanig. Ishke a'aw akiwenziiyiban gii-ikido, ishwaachiwag ingiw Manidoog ekwewijig. Mii a'aw eya'aansiwid ingiw Manidoog ekwewijig a'aw Gaagige-oshkiniigikwe.

[6] Akawe omaa niwii-tibaajimaag ingiw Manidoog ekwewijig, mii inow zeziikizinijin a'aw Wenabozho ogookomisan. Gookomisakiinaan ezhi-wiinind. Gaawiin a'aw akiwenziiyiban ogii-gikenimaasiin gakina ezhi-wiinjigaazonid inow Manidoon ekwewinijin. Mii sa wiin igo aanind ogii-tibaajimaan ezhi-wiinjigaazonid, mii dash a'aw Nabaanaabe, miinawaa a'aw Giganaan a'aw dibiki-giizis, miinawaa aanind ingiw anangoog. Mii a'aw bezhig anang ezhi-wiinind, Nazhike'awaasong.

[4] It is here that I want to talk about the talk that was put in place when a baby is sent off and lost during a woman's pregnancy. What the old men had said was the reason those babies go straight over to where our relatives are, and do not stop here on earth, is that the spirits saw something desirable in that baby, and that is why it was decided they go straight over. When he arrives over there, the spirits will gift the baby with what it is they had in store for that child, and that is the reason why the baby went straight over to where our relatives are to that place called Land of Everlasting Happiness.

[5] There is nothing that those spirits forgot. They also put things in place which will help the babies when it is meant for them to go straight over. The spirit over there that takes care of our relatives has a helper that takes care of the babies. She is known as Forever Young Woman. She is sent here to carry the baby, ensuring that the baby arrives safely over there where our people go. That old man said that there are eight spirits that are women. Forever Young Woman is the youngest of those spirits that are female.

[6] First I am going to tell about the female spirits, the eldest is *Wenabozho*'s grandmother. Her name is Our Grandmother Earth. That old man did not know all the names of the female spirits. He did mention some of them by their names. The Mermaid, and the Moon, and some of the stars. One of the stars' names is The Evening Star—The One That Shines Alone.

[7] Mii omaa akawe nawaj wii-ni-dibaajimoyaan miinawaa. Ishke ingiw abinoojiinyag geshkitoojig babaamibatoowaad omaa akiing gegoo ani-izhiwebiziwaad, mii i'iw bikwaakwad ezhinamowaad i'iw menidoowaadak, mii iw dash beminizha'amowaad imaa miikanensing biinish iwidi ani-dagoshimoonowaad iwidi Gaagige-minawaanigoziwining ezhi-wiinjigaadeg. Mii iw ba-izhinizha'igaadenig i'iw menidoowaadak, mii dash ge-izhinang dibishkoo i'iw bikwaakwad waabandang, mii dash iw nayaanoopinadood biinish iwidi weweni da-ni-dagoshimoonod.

[8] Ishke dash a'aw abinoojiinyens wani'ind dabwaa-wawiinge-giizhigid, gaawiin omaa wiidoopamaasiin omaa dabwaa-maajaa'ind iko endoodawind ani-maajaa'ind nawaj gechi-aya'aawid. Ishke gaa-ikidowaad ingiw akiwenziiyibaneg, gaawiin gii-te-ojichaagoshinziin omaa akiing da-odaapinangiban i'iw wiisiniwin a'aw abinoojiinyens. Gaawiin dash memwech onaagan maagizhaa gaye onaaganan atamawaasiiwag besho enawendaasojig da-ni-wiidoopamaawaad inow neganigowaajin. Mii dash iwidi enabiwaad ingiw Manidoog epagizonjigaadenig i'iw wiisiniwin, mii dash imaa gakina awiya ani-naabishkaaged i'iw wiisiniwin, mii dash iwidi ge-ni-izhaamagak enabiwaad ingiw Manidoog.

[9] Mii gaye ani-bimiwidood a'aw abinoojiinyens i'iw odaminwaagaansi-zhiishiigwan miinawaa i'iw iko eni-noobaajigaadeg omoodens miinawaa doodooshaaboo achigaadeg imaa. Miinawaa iko niminwendaan anishinaabe-zhiiwaagamizigan imaa dagonigaadeg ani-wiishkoba'igaadeg i'iw doodooshaaboo.

[7] It is here I want to tell more. If something happens to a toddler, one that is able to run around on the earth, there is spiritual energy in the form of a ball, and that is what they chase down that path, until they arrive over there to the Land of Everlasting Happiness. It is that spiritual energy that is sent over here that appears in the form of a ball that he sees, that is what he will follow until he arrives safely over there where our relatives are.

[8] If a baby is lost before he is completely developed, we do not eat with these infants before they are sent off like we do with adults. Those old men said that their spirits did not make it to that point where they made an impression on the earth and to be able to accept food. It is not necessary to put a bowl or maybe bowls for the close relatives, since we are not having a meal with the infant. Instead the food is sent over to where the spirits sit, and as everyone eats the food, it in turn goes to where those spirits sit.

[9] The baby will also carry a little toy rattle and a baby bottle filled with milk. I prefer to have people add maple syrup to sweeten the milk.

[10] Mii gaye imaa gashkibijigaazonid inow naaning akeyaa giishkizhigaazonid gendidaawizinijin inow asemaan. Mii inow gendidaawizinijin asemaan iko gaa-shaashaagwamaawaajin ingiw akiwenziiyibaneg miinawaa igo mindimooyenyibaneg. Mii dash i'iw meskwegak gidagiigin, mii imaa gashkibijigaazod a'aw asemaa gaa-kiishkizhigaazod. Meskozid a'aw zenibaanh aabajichigaazod omaa dakobinind a'aw asemaa omaa meskwegak gidagiigin.

[11] Mii iw enaabaji'ind a'aw asemaa, niiwing imaa ani-waawaabanjigaazowag ingiw Manidoog, mii dash ani-biindaakoonindwaa jiigikana naabawijig. Mii dash iwidi ishkwaaj ani-biindaakoonind a'aw Manidoo zhengishing imaa ziibiing iwidi ayaamagak. Mii iko imaa nawaj gechi-aya'aawid inow asemaan imaa baabiitawayi'ii oniibinaakwaanininjiing achigaazonid. Onzaam dash babiiwaamagadiniwan oninjiinsiwaan ingiw biibiiyensag da-achigaazonipan, mii dash i'iw wenji-gashkibijigaazonid inow odasemaawaan.

[12] Gaawiin memwech inow bashkwegino-makizinensan da-biizikoonaasiin a'aw abinoojiinyens. Ishke inow Manidoon inow Gaagige-oshkiniigikwen owii-ni-dakonigoon da-ni-bimiwinigod i'iw miikanensing gaa-miinigoowizid a'aw Anishinaabe da-ni-maada'adood azhigwa gegoo izhiwebizid.

[13] Ishke dash aabiding iwidi maajaa'iweyaan Neyaashiing, mii iw gete-gikinoo'amaadiiwigamig gaa-atemagakiban iko imaa niigaan noongom badakidemagak i'iw ataagewigamig Misi-zaaga'iganiing eyaamagak, mii imaa gaa-tanakamigiziyaang gii-maajaa'ind a'aw abinoojiinyens.

[10] Also a small bundle is made with five pieces of cut-up plug tobacco. That is the kind of tobacco those old men and those old ladies chewed. The cut-up tobacco is then wrapped up in red cloth. A red ribbon is then used to tie up the tobacco in the red cloth.

[11] The purpose of the tobacco is that they will see a spirit on four different occasions; they will offer that tobacco to those spirits who stand alongside that path. The last piece of tobacco is used to offer it to the spirit who is lying in the river that they will come upon. For adults the tobacco is usually put in between their fingers. The hands of an infant are too small to place tobacco; that is why the tobacco is wrapped up in red cloth.

[12] It is not necessary to put moccasins on the infants. The spirit known as Forever Young Woman will carry the infant down that path that the Anishinaabe were given to take when something happens to them.

[13] One time when I was doing a funeral in Mille Lacs, it was in the old schoolhouse that stood in front of where the casino is now in Mille Lacs, it was there that an infant funeral was being held.

[14] Mii dash a'aw abinoojiinyens inow omaamaayan, mii a'aw gii-wiindamaaged gii-waabamaad gii-pi-biindigenid inow Gaagige-oshkiniigikwen iwapii gii-abiichigaazonid inow abinoojiinyensan gaa-wani'aajin. Mii dash gaa-izhinawaad inow Gaagige-oshkiniigikwen, gii-niishtana-biboonagiziwan naa gaye gii-kagaanwaanikwewan, miinawaa gii-makadewaamagadini owiinizisan, mii iwidi gaa-pagamagoodenig owiinizisan imaa odiyaang. Mii dash a'aw ikwe gaa-ikidod, ogii-waabamaan inow Manidoon ganawaabamaanid inow oniijaanisensan. Mii iw gaa-izhi-waabandang i'iw zhawendaagoziwin gaa-ayaamagadinig imaa oshkiinzhigong ganawaabamaad inow oniijaanisensan. Mii-go gaye dibishkoo gaa-izhinamowaad oshkiinzhigong inow oniijaanisensan ganawaabamaad inow Manidoon. Mii dash gaa-ikidod a'aw ikwe, "Mii iw gaa-ondinamaan gaawiin nigagwaadagitoosiin azhigwa gaa-maajaa'ind miinawaa gii-nanaa'inigaazod niniijaanisens."

[14] The infant's mother told about seeing Forever Young Woman come in during the course of the wake. She said Forever Young Woman looked to be about twenty years old and she had long black hair, it hung down to her butt. The mother said she saw that spirit looking at her baby. She saw the compassion of the spirit as she looked at her baby. She could also see the love in the eyes of her baby as he looked back at the spirit. The mother said, "As a result of seeing all this, I did not have a difficult time at the funeral or at the burial of my child."

4 APII GAA-ONDAADIZID

[1] Gaawiin igo aapiji nebowa omaa indayaanziin waa-ni-dazhindamaan apii gaa-ondaadizid a'aw abinoojiinh.

[2] Geget chi-ina'oonwewiziwan iniw ogitiziiman a'aw abinoojiinyens i'iwapii bi-dagoshimoonod. Gayat ingii-tazhindaan iniw Manidoon ogii-inenimigowaan da-miinigoowiziwaad iniw abinoojiinyensan. Ishke gibi-noondaamin iko aanind ingiw abinoojiinyensag ani-inigaachigaazowaad. Ishke ani-inigaachigaazod a'aw abinoojiinyens, mii iniw Manidoon genawenimigojin a'aw abinoojiinyens, mii iniw mayaazhi-doodawiminjin.

[3] Mii dash omaa wii-ni-dazhindamaan iwapii gaa-ondaadiziyaan gaye niin. Ajidiwaashiikwe gii-izhinikaazo niwawiinge-maamaayiban miinawaa niwawiinge-dedeyiban *August Staples* aano-go gii-anishinaabewid, gaawiin ganabaj gii-anishinaabewinikaazosiin.

[4] Ishke dash iwapii gii-ondaadiziyaan gii-shimaaganishiiwi a'aw indedeyiban. Mii dash iwidi agaaming endazhi-miigaading gii-maakishkoozod. Mii imaa oshtigwaaning gii-maakishkoozod.

[5] Ishke dash gii-pi-giiwed, ingii-abinoojiinyensiw. Mii dash a'aw nimaamaayiban gaa-ikidod gii-mawiyaan ogii-gotaan da-wanishkwe'igod indedeyiban. Gaawiin weweni gii-izhi-ayaasiin omaa naanaagadawendamowining a'aw indedeyiban. Mii imaa gaa-onjikaamagadinig gii-maakishkoozod.

4 AT THE TIME OF THE BIRTH OF A CHILD

[1] I do not have a lot to talk about when it comes to the birth of a child.

[2] It is a special gift to the parents when a child is born and comes into their life. I had mentioned earlier where the spirits intended that these parents be given this child. We have heard in the past where children were abused. When a child is harmed, the spirits that take care of this child are directly harmed.

[3] It is at this time I am going to talk about my upbringing. My biological mother, her name was Nancy Churchill, and my biological father August Staples; even though he was Anishinaabe, I do not think he had an Anishinaabe name.

[4] At the time that I was born my father was in the armed services. While he was overseas during the war, he was wounded. He was shot in the head.

[5] When he came home, I was a baby. My mother said that she was afraid that the noise of my crying would disturb my father. My father's mental state was not quite right. It was a result of his war injury.

[6] Mii dash i'iw gii-niiwo-giiziswagiziyaan, mii iwapii nimaamaayiban gii-inendang a'aw ninoshenh da-ganawenimid. Mii dash a'aw Nazhikewigaabawiikweban miinawaa Ogimaawabiban gii-maajii-ganawenimiwaad. Geget ingii-mino-doodaagoog. Ishke mii eta-go gii-anishinaabemowaad. Gaawiin gii-nitaa-zhaaganaashiimosiiwag miinawaa mii-go apane gii-ayaangwaamitoowaad gaa-izhi-miinigoowiziyang anishinaabewiyang. Ogii-kanawenimaan iniw Manidoo-dewe'iganan a'aw akiwenziiyiban miinawaa mii imaa gii-naadamaagewaad Anishinaaben midewinid, miinawaa a'aw mindimooyenyiban nebowa ogii-gikendaanan mashkikiwan imaa wendinigaadenig imaa bagwaj.

[7] Ishke dash mii imaa wenjikaamagak nitaa-ojibwemoyaan miinawaa wiikwajitooyaan ani-ayaangwaamitooyaan gaa-izhi-miinigoowiziyang anishinaabewiyang. Ishke giishpin gii-ni-aabiji-wiij'ayaawagwaaban dedebinawe nigitiziimag, gaawiin indaa-gii-gikendanziin da-ojibwemoyaan miinawaa da-ni-ganoodamawag Anishinaabe ani-asemaaked.

[8] Ishke ingiw dedebinawe niwiij'aya'aag, gaawiin nitaa-ojibwemosiiwag miinawaa aanind ogii-mamoonaawaa i'iw wayaabishkiiwen ezhitwaanid. Ganabaj ingii-inendaagoz omaa da-ni-wiij'ayaawagwaa ingiw gechi-aya'aawijig da-ni-gikendamaan dash i'iw Ojibwemowin miinawaa eni-izhichiged a'aw Anishinaabe eni-asemaaked. Mii dash o'ow noongom wendinamaan ani-naadamawag niwiiji-anishinaabem.

[6] I was four months old when my mother decided that my aunt should take care of me. That is when Sophia Churchill and John Benjamin took me in. They were good to me. They only spoke Ojibwe. They did not know how to speak English, and they were always in and around those ceremonies we were given as a people. That old man took care of a ceremonial drum, they helped the Anishinaabe with the Midewiwin ceremony, and that old lady knew medicines that you could pick from the wild.

[7] It is the reason that I am fluent in Ojibwe, and it is from there that my desire to concentrate on our ceremonies that we were given as a people comes from. If I had to continue to stay with my biological parents, I would not have known the Ojibwe language and have the ability to speak for Anishinaabe as they put out their tobacco.

[8] My biological brothers and sisters are not able to speak the Ojibwe language, and some of them have converted to Christianity. I believe it was meant for me to live with these old people so that I would be able to speak the language and know these ceremonies where Anishinaabe offer their tobacco. It is from there that I have the capability to help my fellow Anishinaabe.

5 ASABIKESHIINH-WANII'IGAN

[1] Mii dash omaa waa-ni-dazhindamaan i'iw asabikeshiinh-wanii'igan iko gaa-agoojigaadenig omaa odikinaaganing ingiw giniijaanisinaanig. Mii o'ow asabikeshiinh-wanii'igan wenji-wiindamaan iniw, mii iw ezhinaagwak. Mii ingiw mindimooyenyibaneg gaa-ikidowaad, gaawiin gii-ayaamagasinoon gaa-izhi-anishinaabewinikaadeg iniw. Niin igo nimichi-giizhitoon. Mii dash gaa-inaabadadinig a'aw abinoojiinyens eta-go wenaajiwaninig akeyaa da-izhingwashid. Mii dash i'iw iko awiya zegingwashid, mii imaa ani-baataasininig imaa egoojigaadenig odikinaaganing. Mii dash gaawiin da-zegingwashisiin a'aw abinoojiinyens. Mii dash i'iw enaabadak.

[2] Mii iw wayeshkad gaa-onji-miinigoowiziyang iniw asabikeshiinh-wanii'iganan ezhinaagwakin da-naadamaagod a'aw abinoojiinyens eta-go wenaajiwaninig akeyaa da-inaabandang. Ishke dash i'iw noongom niwaabandaanan anooj inaabadak iniw. Wawaaj igo biinji-odaabaan agoojigaadewanoon. Maagizhaa gaye wii-zazegaatood imaa endaad a'aw bemaadizid, mii imaa aasamisagong wawaaj egoojigaadenig iniw.

[3] Gaawiin gidaa-wii-baapinendanziimin gaa-izhi-miinigoowiziyang anishinaabewiyang. Gaawiin i'iw anooj daa-inaabadasinoon iniw Manidoo-aabajichiganan gaa-miinigoowiziyang anishinaabewiyang. Ishke mii imaa wanitood a'aw bemaadizid i'iw wayeshkad gaa-izhi-gikinoo'amaagoowiziyang da-inaabadak iniw asabikeshiinh-wanii'iganan. Mii i'iw wayaabishkiiwed ezhi-wiindang *Dream-catcher*.

5 DREAM CATCHERS

[1] What I want to talk about are the dream catchers that were hung on the cradleboards of our babies. The reason I call them spider webs is because that is what they look like. Those old ladies had said there was not an Anishinaabe name for those dream catchers. I was the one who created that name for them. It was used to help the baby to have only good dreams. When someone is having bad dreams, the bad dream gets stuck in the dream catcher that is hanging on their cradleboard. So as a result the child or baby will not have bad dreams. That is how the dream catchers are used.

[2] We were originally given the dream catchers to help filter the baby's dreams so that the baby will only have good dreams. Now-adays I see dream catchers used in different ways. They are even hung inside of cars. People are even using them as decoration placed on the walls of their homes.

[3] We should not disrespect those things that were given to us as Anishinaabe. We should not use our spiritual items that were given to us as Anishinaabe in ways that were not intended. This is where Anishinaabe have lost the original teaching of how to use a dream catcher. This is what the white man calls a dream catcher.

6 BASHKWEGINO-MAKIZINENSAN A'AW ABINOOJIINYENS

[1] Ishke wayeshkad ozhitamawaad bashkwegino-makizinensan iniw abinoojiinyensan a'aw Anishinaabe, mii iw ezhichigaadang iniw bashkwegino-makizinensan, mii imaa bapagone'ang imaa onagaakizidaang iniw bashkwegino-makizinensan. Mii dash iw wenji-izhichigaadang a'aw Anishinaabe, owaabandaanaawaa ingiw abinoojiinyensag gakina gegoo wawaaj igo Manidoon.

[2] Bagakendamoog, mii iw wenji-waabandamowaad gakina gegoo wawaaj igo iniw Manidoon bimi-ayaanid. Nawaj gechi-aya'aawijig nebowa odayaanaawaa imaa odinendamowiniwaa wenishkwe'igowaad. Gaawiin wiinawaa gakina gegoo owaabandanziinaawaa dibishkoo iniw abinoojiinyensan waabandaminid.

[3] Ishke dash awiya apii ishkwaa-ayaad, mii imaa ganawenjigaazod niiwo-dibik dabwaa-na'inigaazod. Mii dash owapii babaamaadizinid iniw ojichaagwan baa-mawidisaadaminid aaniindi-go gii-pabaa-ayaanid megwaa maa gii-pibizhaagiinid omaa akiing. Ishke dash bimi-ayaanid ojichaagwan awiya maagizhaa gaye iniw Manidoon besho imaa ayaad a'aw abinoojiinyens, mii dash ge-izhi-wiindamawaad omaa bemi-ayaanijin. "Gaawiin gidaa-ni-wiijiiwisinoon, onzaam bapagoshkaamagadoon nimbashkwegino-makizinensan." Mii iw epenimod a'aw Anishinaabe weweni da-izhi-ayaanid oniijaanisensan.

6 A CHILD'S FIRST MOCCASINS

[1] When Anishinaabe make the baby's first pair of moccasins, this is what is done with those moccasins: he makes small holes on the soles of the moccasins. The reason why Anishinaabe make the moccasins this way is because babies are able to see everything including spirits.

[2] Their minds are clear; that is why they are able to see everything, even the spirits as they go by. Those who are older have a lot on their minds that distract them. Therefore they are not able to see everything that a baby is able to see.

[3] When someone passes on they are kept over for four nights before burial. It is at that time that the spirit of the individual travels and revisits every place they had been while they lived on this earth. When the spirit of the individual is traveling by, or maybe a spirit gets close to where that baby is, the baby speaks out and says, "I cannot travel with you, because my moccasins have holes in them." This is what Anishinaabe rely on to ensure their baby's safety.

7 OSHKI-DAANGISHKANG I'IW AKI A'AW ABINOOJIINYENS

[1] Azhigwa gaa-niiwo-giizhigadinig owapii gaa-ondaadizid a'aw abinoojiinyens, mii iniw ogitiziiman ezhi-zagaswe'idinid iniw asemaan miinawaa wiisiniwin atamawaawaad iniw Manidoon ge-onjikaamagadinig da-ni-naadamaagoowizinid inow oniijaanisiwaan oniigaaniiming.

[2] Ishke minochige a'aw Anishinaabe gaabige iniw asemaan miinawaa wiisiniwin ani-atamawaad iniw oniijaanisensan weweni dash da-ni-gikenimigod iniw Manidoon awenen aawid. Mii imaa ani-miigwechiwi'indwaa ingiw Manidoog weweni gii-pi-dagoshimoononid iniw oniijaanisensan miinawaa weweni ani-izhi-ayaanid iniw omaamaayan. Mii gaye omaa anamikawind a'aw abinoojiinyens.

[3] Mii dash iwidi eni-apagizondamawindwaa ingiw Manidoog enabiwaad iniw asemaan miinawaa i'iw wiisiniwin ani-miigwechiwi'indwaa ingiw Manidoog imaa ani-oshki-dagoshimoononid iniw oniijaanisensan. Mii gaye omaa ge-ondiniged a'aw abinoojiinyens mino-ayaawin da-ni-miinigoowizid oniigaaniiming miinawaa iniw Manidoon weweni da-ni-ganawenimigod. Mii gaye imaa nandodamaageng da-wawiingezinid iniw ogitiziiman da-ni-ganawenimigod oniigaaniiming da-ni-manezisinig gegoo miinawaa da-ni-mino-doodaagod.

7 WHEN A CHILD FIRST TOUCHES THE GROUND

[1] On the fourth day following the birth of a child, his or her parents give a feast in which tobacco and food is offered up for the spirits; it is from there that their baby will be helped in his or her future.

[2] Anishinaabe do good by putting tobacco and food for their baby; as a result those spirits will know who their baby is. It is then that appreciation is expressed for the safe arrival of their baby, and also for the well-being of the mother. This is the time the baby is being welcomed into the world.

[3] The tobacco and food is offered to the spirits for the recent arrival of their baby. It is from here that the baby is given good health, and also that spirits will take good care of the child in the future. It is also at this time that it is asked that the parents do a real good job in taking care of this child in their future, that the parents are not without, and also that they treat the baby in a good way.

[4] Azhigwa dash ani-giizhiitaang ani-naabishkaageng i'iw wiisiniwin eninamawindwaa ingiw Manidoog, mii dash agwajiing ezhiwinind a'aw abinoojiinyens, mii dash imaa oshki-daangishkang i'iw aki. Mii dash imaa gaye ani-ojichaagoshing omaa akiing a'aw abinoojiinyens, mii iw ingiw akiwenziiyibaneg gaa-izhi-wiindamowaad.

[5] Mii imaa mitadaawangaanig daangizideshimoono'ind atamawind ozidensan a'aw abinoojiinyens. Akawe sa wiin igo asemaa achigaazo omaa mitadaawangaag, mii dash imaa ozidensan atamawind a'aw abinoojiinyens. Giishpin biboong booch da-mangaanibiing da-ni-moonikeng imaa dabazhish da-ayaamagak dash imaa mitadaawangaanig da-ni-daangizideshkang i'iw aki a'aw abinoojiinyens.

[6] Mewinzha a'aw Anishinaabe gii-wenipanizi gii-ayaad imaa wiigiwaaming megwe-bibooninig. Gaawiin memwech imaa agwajiing gii-izhiwijigaazosiin a'aw abinoojiinyens. Mii-go imaa biinji-wiigiwaam gii-oshki-daangishkang i'iw aki a'aw abinoojiinyens.

[4] When the feast is finished and the food has been handed to the spirits, the baby is taken outside, and their feet will touch the earth for the first time. It is then that their spirit will make its first impression on the earth, as those old men refer to it.

[5] The baby's little feet are placed directly on the ground in the dirt. First tobacco is placed in the dirt, and then the baby's little feet are placed on the ground. If it is winter, shoveling has to be done to uncover the bare ground below in order for the baby to touch its feet to the ground.

[6] It was much easier for Anishinaabe long ago, since they lived in wigwams. They did not have to take the baby outside. The baby was able to complete the welcoming ceremony inside their wigwams.

8 ODISIINS

[1] I'iwapii oshki-ondaadizid a'aw abinoojiinyens, odayaan imaa omigiid imaa odisiinsing. Azhigwa dash bakwajisemagadinig imaa omigiid imaa odisiinsing, mii i'iw omigiiwin genawenjigaadenig. Mii imaa mashkimodensing achigaadenig miinawaa asemaa. Mii dash a'aw Anishinaabe gaa-izhi-wiindang odisiins a'aw abinoojiinyens. Mii-go gaa-izhi-aabiji-ganawendang o'ow odisiins a'aw Anishinaabe. Ishke dash owapii gii-ni-ishkwaa-ayaad a'aw Anishinaabe, mii-go gii-ni-maajiidood o'ow odisiins.

[2] Ishke dash ezhiwebizid iko a'aw Anishinaabe nandawaabandang gegoo anooj nandobijiged, mii-ko dash wawiyazh ani-gagwejimind awiya, "Awegonen danaa nendawaabandaman? Mii na iw gidisiins nendawaabandaman?"

8 A CHILD'S BELLY BUTTON

[1] At the time of birth a baby has a small scab on their belly button. Once that scab falls off of their belly button, it is that scab that is kept. It is put into a little bag with tobacco. That is what Anishinaabe call a belly button. Anishinaabe always held on to that belly button. At the time of death, Anishinaabe took their belly button with them.

[2] When an Anishinaabe has lost something and is forever looking around for it, they are jokingly asked, "What are you looking for? Are you looking for your belly button?"

9 WIIYAWEN'ENYIKAAGENG/
WIINDAAWASONG

[1] Mii dash i'iw wiiyawen'enyikaageng waa-ni-dazhindamaan. Wewiib igo daa-miinaa a'aw abinoojiinyens da-anishinaabewinikaazod. Giishpin wewiib miinaasiwind da-anishinaabewinikaazod, daa-mawi moozhag a'aw abinoojiinyens. Mii iw wenji-mawid misawendang miinawaa nandwewendang da-anishinaabewinikaazod.

[2] Mii dash iniw ogitiziiman da-onaabamaanid ge-wiiyawen'enyinijin iniw oniijaanisiwaan. Mii-go a'aw abinoojiinyens odedeyan, mii-go dibishkoo minik ge-onaabamaanid minik ge-onaabamaanid iniw omaamaayan waa-wiiyawen'enyinijin. Ishke iniw odedeyan niizh onaabamaanid, mii-go gaye a'aw abinoojiinyens iniw omaamaayan niizh da-onaabamaanid.

[3] Gego nebowa odaa-onaabamaasiwaawaan. Odaa-wii-mikwendaanaawaa inow waa-kanoodamaagowaajin booch da-dazhimaad gakina bebezhig odasemaawaan naa wiisiniwin waa-atamawaawaad waa-onaabamaawaajin. Ginwenzh imaa da-ni-gaagiigido giishpin nebowa inow wiiyawen'enyan miinaawaad inow oniijaanisiwaan.

9 GIVING A BABY NAMESAKES/NAMING CEREMONY

[1] I want to talk about the namesake ceremony. A name should be given to a child as soon as possible. If a child is not given an Anishinaabe name right away, that baby might cry often. The reason a child cries is that he is expressing the desire and need to have an Anishinaabe name.

[2] It is the parents that will select the individuals that will be namesakes to their child. Both the father and the mother of that child should both pick an equal number of namesakes that they want for their child. If the father picks two, the mother should also pick two.

[3] They should not pick too many namesakes. They should remember the one who is speaking has to talk for each individual's tobacco and food that they will put for the namesakes. The speaker will be talking for a good length of time if there are many namesakes chosen for the child.

[4] Ishke aabiding gii-kanoodamaageyaan gii-wiiyawen'enyikaageng, niishtana ogii-onaabamaawaan, ginwenzh dash ingii-ni-gaagiigid. Gii-onzaamichigewag. Mii imaa niishtana onaaganan gii-ateg imaa ogijayi'ii anaakaning gaa-aabajitooyaang. Ishke dash a'aw Gete-anishinaabe imaa gii-ayaapan, daa-gii-maamakaadendam naa gaye daa-gii-wenda-biingeyendam waabandangiban imaa gaa-izhichigeng. Miinawaa mewinzha gakina ingiw gaa-onaabaminjig gii-kanoodamaadizowag. Aaniish naa gakina ogii-gikendaanaawaa Ojibwemowin i'iwapii.

[5] Ishke dash ingiw Anishinaabebaneg gaa-inaawaad iniw ogitiziiman a'aw abinoojiinyens, moozhag mikwenimeg awiya ge-wiiyawen'enyikawind, gego zhiigwaakonaakegon. Mii-go ge-izhi-gikendang a'aw abinoojiinyens. Mii-go moozhag ge-izhi-mawid. Misawaa-go giiwashkwebiishkid maagizhaa gaye gagiibaadizid a'aw mekwenimind, mii-go booch da-onaabamind da-wiiyawen'enyikawind iniw abinoojiinyensan. Misawaa-go eni-inaadizid omaa akiing awiya, weweni-go izhi-ayaawan inow ojichaagwan.

[6] Ishke dash noongom ezhichigewaad ingiw Anishinaabeg, mii-go biinizikaa ezhi-miinaawaad iniw abinoojiinyensan ge-izhinikaazonid. Ishke bezhig a'aw mindimooyenh ingii-noondawaa, mii iw gaa-inaad iniw abinoojiinyensan, "Giwii-kinooz, mii iw Zhingwaak waa-miininaan da-izhinikaazoyan." Weweni-go nigii-wiindamawaa a'aw mindimooyenh, "Gaawiin gidaa-izhichigesiin i'iw. Gaawiin i'iw akeyaa gigii-izhi-gikinoo'amaagoowizisiimin anishinaabewiyang." Gego daa-wii-izhichigesiin awiya i'iw akeyaa. Booch iniw Manidoon da-gii-shawenimigod da-gii-waabanda'igoowizid gegoo imaa bawaajiganing. Mii imaa wendinang wiindaawasod a'aw Anishinaabe.

[4] This one time that I was speaking at this namesake ceremony, and there were twenty namesakes that were selected for that child, and I talked for a long time to cover each and every one of them. They got carried away. We had twenty dishes on the mat that was being used. If Anishinaabe from long ago were present there, they would have been baffled and dumbfounded if they saw what was being done at this ceremony. And also a long time ago each of those selected as namesakes were able to talk for themselves. Everybody knew the language at that time.

[5] Anishinaabe in the past have said to the parents of the child, if an individual comes to mind frequently as a namesake to your child, make sure you select them. The child will know if you rule them out. The baby will cry a lot as a result. If that person that is being considered is a drunk or is foolish, be sure to select them anyway to be a namesake to that child. No matter how someone conducts themselves on this earth, their spirit is pure.

[6] What a lot of our Anishinaabe are doing today, just out of the clear blue they will give an Anishinaabe name to the baby. I overheard this old lady telling that child that was about to be given a name, "I am going to give you the name White Pine, because you are going to be tall when you get older." I told the old lady, "You cannot do that. We were not taught to do that as Anishinaabe." Nobody should do that. In order to give a name the spirits will have to have shown him or her something in a dream or vision. It is from there, from what they have been shown, that they give the child an Anishinaabe name.

[7] Ishke aanind owaabandaanaawaa gegoo. Ishke a'aw bezhig niitaawis ogii-waabamaan iniw bagwaj-ininiwan. Mii imaa wendinang miinaad iniw abinoojiinyensan ge-izhinikaazonid. Ishke booch imaa da-ayaamagadinig gegoo gaa-miinigoowizid imaa bawaajiganing maagizhaa gaye ogii-michi-waabamaan iniw Manidoon megwaa baa-ayaad omaa akiing. Mii imaa wendinang i'iw izhinikaazowin maanaad iniw abinoojiinyensan.

[8] Mii inow odasemaan miinawaa wiisiniwin enikaamagadinig inow Manidoon gaa-pi-zhawenimigojin nanaandomaad idash aazhita da-zhawenimaad inow gaa-oshki-wiiyawen'enyikawiminjin. Ishke dash ingiw Manidoog ominwendaanaawaa noondamowaad ezhinikaazonid inow Anishinaabe-abinoojiinyan. Aaniish naa mii iw iwidi gaa-onjikaamagadinig imaa apinikaazod iniw Manidoon gaa-shawenimigojin a'aw waandaawasod. Ishke iko noondamaan anooj ezhinikaazowaad ingiw Anishinaabeg, mii imaa wiindamaagoowiziyaan ezhi-chi-manidoowaadadinig enaabandang a'aw Anishinaabe.

[9] Ishke a'aw Anishinaabe biinizikaa ani-miinaad inow abinoojiinyan ge-izhinikaazonid ayaanzig i'iw gaa-izhingwashid inow Manidoon gii-pi-zhawenimigod maagizhaa gaye gaawiin ogii-waabamaasiin inow Manidoon, gaawiin imaa da-ayaamagasinini a'aw abinoojiinh ge-ondiniged da-ni-maajiikamigaanig i'iw aki da-ni-naadamaagoowizid.

[10] Booch a'aw waandaawasod da-ayaawaad inow Manidoon gaa-pi-zhawenimigojin. Mii dash inow nenaandomaajin aazhita da-zhawenimaanid inow oshki-wiiyawen'enyan. Ishke mii iw gaawiin imaa da-ayaamagasinini iko anooj izhichiged a'aw Anishinaabe biinizikaa inendaagwadinig baa-waawiindaawasod.

[7] See, some of our Anishinaabe have seen things. One of my close relatives had seen that man that lives in the wild. It is from there that he gives Anishinaabe names to babies. The one who gives a name has to have been shown something in their dreams by the spirits, or they see them in the flesh while they were out and about. It is from there that they get the name that they give to a child.

[8] The tobacco given to them and the food before them will go to that spirit that took pity on them, asking that same spirit in turn to have compassion for their new namesake. The spirits like to hear the name that was given to the child. After all, the name came from them originally when they gifted that person with a dream or showed them something. When I hear the Anishinaabe names that some of our people have been given I realize what a gift that name giver must have been shown by those spirits.

[9] If an Anishinaabe gives a name out of the clear blue without having a dream where those spirits came forward and took pity on them, or did not see a spirit in the physical world, the child will not be provided with this spiritual support in their future that comes from an Anishinaabe who knows what he is doing when he is giving a name.

[10] The one who is giving a name has to have a spirit that took pity on him. It is that spirit that he calls on to in turn also to give spiritual support to his new namesake. That will be missing for a child that is being given a name by someone who does not know what he or she is doing.

[11] Ishke gaye noongom geget anooj izhichige a'aw
Anishinaabe. Mii-go aaningodinong ani-noondamaan
anishinaabewinikaazowinan, mii-go ezhi-gikendamaan, gaawiin
nitaawichigesiin, maagizhaa gaye gaawiin nitaa-ojibwemosiin
gaa-miigiwed i'iw izhinikaazowin. Aanind a'aw Anishinaabe
wenda-gagwaadaginikaazo noongom.

[12] Giishpin imaa ayaasig gaa-miinigoowizid da-wiindaawasod,
mii-go bezhig a'aw gaa-wiiyawen'enyikawind ge-izhi-miinaapan
iniw abinoojiinyensan odizhinikaazowin. Ishke a'aw bezhig
a'aw inini ge-wiiyawen'enyikawind, odaa-miinaan iniw
gwiiwizensan odizhinikaazowin. Mii-go gaye ge-izhichigepan
a'aw ikwe ge-wiiyawen'enyikawind, mii-go ge-izhi-miinaapan
inow ikwezensan ge-wiiyawen'enyikawimind wiin igo
odizhinikaazowin gaa-miinigoowizid.

[13] Ishke i'iwapii gii-wiiyawen'enyikaagooyaan, gii-niiwiwag
ingiw niiyawen'enyag. Gaawiin dash gii-miinigoowizisiiwag
da-wiindaawasowaad. Mii dash a'aw zeziikizid a'aw
akiwenziiyiban gaa-wiiyawen'enyiyaan, mii a'aw gaa-miizhid
indizhinikaazowin. Mii dash i'iw Obizaan wenji-izhinikaazoyaan
noongom. Obizaanigiizhig gii-izhinikaazo a'aw akiwenziiyiban.

[14] Ishke dash omaa niwii-ni-dazhindaan i'iw zagaswe'iding apii
wiiyawen'enyikaageng. Gaawiin eta-go anishinaabewinikaazowin
miinigoowizisiin a'aw abinoojiinyens. Mii gaye imaa ani-
miinigoowizid ge-ni-naadamaagod oniigaaniiming.

[11] Our Anishinaabe people do a lot of foolish things today. As I go about and hear some of the Anishinaabe names that our people have, it is clear to me that the particular name giver did not know what he was doing or did not know our language very well. Some of our Anishinaabe have screwed-up names nowadays.

[12] If there is no one there that has been given the gift to give Anishinaabe names, one of the namesakes that was selected can give the child his or her name. One of the male namesakes can give his Anishinaabe name to the little boy, and one of the women selected as a namesake can give her Anishinaabe name to a baby girl.

[13] At the namesake ceremony for me, I had four namesakes that were selected. The namesakes of mine were never given the ability to give names. The eldest old man that was chosen as one of my namesakes gave me his Anishinaabe name. That is why I have the name *Obizaan,* which was the name that old man had. The old man's name was *Obizaanigiizhig.*

[14] At this time I want to talk about the feast that is given when the child is given namesakes. At that time, a child is not only given an Anishinaabe name, but also given spiritual support to help him in his future.

[15] Booch weweni asemaan weniijaanisijig da-miinaawaad gaa-onaabamaawaajin da-wiiyawen'enyinid iniw oniijaanisensiwaan. Mii dash imaa onabi'indwaa ingiw ge-wiiyawen'enyikawinjig. Mii dash a'aw abinoojiinh inow odedeyan maagizhaa inow omaamaayan ge-izhi-onabi'aanid gaa-onaabamaanijin, da-niibidebi'aanid, mii dash gaye wiinitam awedi bezhig a'aw abinoojiinh ogitiziiman da-niibidebi'aanid gaye wiin gaa-mikwenimaanijin.

[16] Mii dash imaa wiisiniwin achigaadenig enaasamabiwaad ingiw ge-wiiyawen'enyikawinjig. Mii dash inow wededeyijin baa-ininamawaad oniijaanisensan iniw gaa-onaabamaajin, mii dash enaad, "Gimiinin nigozis/nindaanis da-wiiyawen'enyiyan". Mii dash inow wemaamaayijin a'aw abinoojiinyens, mii gaye gakina eni-doodawaanid gaa-onaabamaanijin da-wiiyawen'enyinid oniijaanisensan. Mii dash a'aw ge-wiiyawen'enyikawind, mii maa minik omaa ani-dakonaad iniw abinoojiinyensan miinawaa ojiimaad.

[17] Ishke dash noongom eshkam nebowa ayaa a'aw Anishinaabe netaa-ojibwemosig. Mii dash imaa ani-ganoodamawagwaa gakina. Ishke dash ezhi-gikinoo'amaagooyang anishinaabewiyang, gakina a'aw Anishinaabe odayaawaan iniw Manidoon zhewenimigojin. Gaawiin omaa daa-ayaasiin omaa akiing ayaawaasig.

[15] The parents of the child will have to offer their tobacco to the namesakes they have selected for their child. The namesakes that were selected are seated in a particular order. Then the child's father or maybe the mother seats the ones they have chosen next to each other, and then the other parent also does the same by seating the ones they have selected next to each other.

[16] Plates of food are put before the namesakes. Then the father takes his child and hands him to each of the namesakes he selected and says to them, "I give you my son/daughter to be your namesake." The mother does likewise to all the namesakes that she has selected for their child. All the namesakes that are present will hold the baby for a little bit and give them a kiss.

[17] Today there are more and more Anishinaabe that do not know our language. When I speak for all of the namesakes, I offer up all the tobacco and the food to the spirits that take care of them. Our teaching is that each of us as Anishinaabe have spirits that watch over us. Anishinaabe would not be on this earth without a spirit watching over them.

[18] Mii dash omaa ani-dazhimag a'aw asemaa gaa-miinindwaa miinawaa wiisiniwin gaa-achigaadenig enaasamabiwaad ingiw gaa-onaabaminjig da-wiiyawen'enyiwaad iniw abinoojiinyensan. Mii dash imaa asemaan miinawaa wiisiniwin iwidi ani-apagizondamawagwaa ingiw Manidoog genawenimigowaajin bebezhig ingiw ge-wiiyawen'enyikawinjig nanaandomagwaa ingiw Manidoog aazhita gaye da-ni-ganawenimaawaad iniw weshki-wiiyawen'enyikawiminjin. Mii-go gaye iwidi ani-apagizomag a'aw asemaa miinawaa wiisiniwin iniw Manidoon epinikaazowaad ingiw ge-wiiyawen'enyikawinjig.

[19] Mii dash imaa gaye niin ani-dazhimag a'aw asemaa maagizhaa gaye odedeyan maagizhaa gaye iniw omaamaayan ogii-mooshkina'aan inow indoopwaaganan. Mii dash omaa ani-apagizomag a'aw asemaa miinawaa wiisiniwin iwidi ingiw Manidoog gaa-pi-zhawenimijig. Mii dash imaa dibaajimoyaan weweni gaa-izhingwashiyaan. Mii dash imaa da-ni-wiindamaageyaan gaa-waabanda'igoowiziyaan miinawaa gaa-inaabamagwaa ingiw Manidoog gii-pawaajigeyaan. Mii dash imaa wendinamaan miinag a'aw abinoojiinyens ge-izhinikaazod. Mii dash gaye nanaandomagwaa ingiw Manidoog dibishkoo da-ni-zhawenimaawaad iniw abinoojiinyensan weshki-wiiyawen'enyikaagooyaan.

[20] Mii dash gaye imaa naawayi'ii atemagak i'iw wiisiniwin, mii imaa wiigwaas-asemaa-onaagan achigaadeg. Mii dash gaye omaa odasemaawaan biinjina asaanid iniw ogitiziiman a'aw abinoojiinyens. Mii imaa da-ni-dazhimag a'aw asemaa gaye. Mii dash gaye i'iw wiisiniwin omaa booch atemagadogwen gaa-ishkosenig gaa-ni-giizhiitaang i'iw wiisiniwin gii-atamawindwaa ge-wiiyawen'enyikawinjig.

[18] As I speak for each of the namesakes, I offer the tobacco given to them and the food put before them, asking those spirits that have watched over them in their lives and asking that in turn they also watch over their new namesake they are being given in this ceremony. Each of them chosen as namesakes also have an Anishinaabe name that was given to them and came from the spirits; I also offer the tobacco and food to those particular spirits that their names are based on.

[19] I then speak for the tobacco that has been put in my pipe by either the mother or the father or both. I offer the tobacco and food to those spirits that took pity on me in my dreams. It is there that I give the details surrounding the dream that I was given. I then tell what was shown or felt in those dreams. It is from there that I give the child his name. I ask those spirits to watch over that child that I have been given as a new namesake.

[20] There is a small birch bark basket that has been put in the middle of the food before us. The parents also put tobacco in that small birch bark basket. I also speak for that tobacco. There is also probably food that was left over after the plates of food were set out for the namesakes.

[21] Mii dash inow odasemaawaan naa i'iw wiisiniwin ani-apagizondamawagwaa ingiw Manidoog enabiwaad. Mii dash imaa oshki-noondamowaad ingiw Manidoog ezhinikaazonid inow abinoojiinyensan. Gaawiin wiikaa oga-wanenimigoosiin awenen aawid a'aw abinoojiinyens.

[22] Mii dash imaa wenaajiwaninig nandodamaageyaan da-miinigoowizid a'aw niiyawen'enh mino-ayaawin, mino-mamaajiiwin, miinawaa da-naadamaagoowizid azhigwa gikinoo'amaagozid. Mii imaa ge-ondiniged da-ni-bami'idizod oniigaaniiming.

[23] Mii gaye imaa nandodamaageyaan a'aw niiyawen'enh oga-wenda-gikendaan gaa-izhi-miinigoowizid a'aw Anishinaabe. Mii imaa ge-ondiniged da-ni-baazhidaakonigoowizid imaa oniigaaniiming.

[24] Mii gaye nanaandomagwaa ingiw Binesiwag weweni da-bimi-ayaawaad aaniindi-go da-baa-ayaad niiyawen'enh. Mii gaye iwidi ani-apagizondamawagwaa ingiw Manidoog imaa eyaajig ziibiing miinawaa zaaga'iganiing weweni da-ganawenjigaazod a'aw niiyawen'enh aaniin igo apii da-baa-ayaad omaa nibiikaang. Weweni da-ganawenjigaazod omaa baa-odaminod imaa nibiikaang, maagizhaa gaye baa-wewebanaabiid, miinawaa baa-manoominiked, biinish igo gaye aaniin igo apii waa-paa-bagida'waad. Gego da-wii-maazhisesiin baa-ayaad imaa nibiikaang. Weweni iniw Manidoon imaa nibiikaang odaa-wii-kanawenimigoon.

[25] Biinish gaye mii imaa ge-inikaad a'aw asemaa miinawaa i'iw wiisiniwin omaa Manidoo omaa akiing eyaad. Weweni dash daa-wii-ganawenjigaazo a'aw niiyawen'enh omaa babaamibatood miinawaa babaa-odaminod omaa akiing.

[21] It is then that I offer up the tobacco and the food to the spirits where they sit. It is then that the spirits first hear the Anishinaabe name given to the child. From there on out the spirits will never forget who the child is.

[22] It is there that I ask for the good things are given to my new namesake such as good health, good movement, and to be given help when the child begins to go to school. It is from that schooling that they will be given the ability to support himself or herself in the future.

[23] I also ask at that time that my new namesake is able to learn the Anishinaabe way of life that we have been given. It is from those teachings that the child will be given the ability to get over hurdles in his or her life.

[24] I also ask the Thunder-beings go over carefully wherever my namesake may be. I also offer up the food and tobacco to those spirits in the rivers and the lakes so that he or she is taken care of whenever he or she is in or around the water. I ask that the child be watched over when playing in the water, when out fishing, out harvesting wild rice, and even when the child is out setting nets. I ask that nothing bad happen to the child when he or she is out and about in the water. I ask those spirits that are in the lakes and rivers to take good care of my namesake.

[25] I offer the tobacco and food to the spirit in the earth. I ask that they watch over my namesake while he or she plays on this earth.

[26] Manidoog ayaawag wenjida zhewinimaajig inow Anishinaabe-abinoojiinyan. Apane-go ingii-pi-noondaan, mii iniw Manidoon gaa-pi-wiiji'igowaajin ingiw gidanishinaabe-abinoojiinyiminaanig. Mii dash ingiw Memengwesiwag miinawaa Manidoo-gwiiwizensag iko ezhi-wiinjigaazojig gaye. Mii dash iwidi apagizondamawagwaa inow asemaan naa wiisiniwin weweni da-ganawenimaawaad niiyawen'enyiminaanin.

[27] Mii-ko gaye omaa nandodamaageyaan da-naadamaagoowizid a'aw niiyawen'enh oniigaaniiming da-ni-bitaakoshkanzig i'iw waabandanziwang aakoziwin ezhi-wiinjigaadeg. Mii gaye waa-izhichigeyaan niwii-nanaandonge ingiw niiyawen'enyag da-maamiijiwaad i'iw wiisiniwin ge-minokaagowaad. Ishke noongom a'aw Anishinaabe omaamiijin i'iw wiisiniwin wenjikaamagadinig anooj inaapined ziinzibaakwadwaapined, maagizhaa gaye ishpiming izhaamagadinig omiskwiim, maagizhaa gaye gegoo izhiwebizid imaa ode'ing.

[28] Mii gaye waa-kagwedweyaan da-naadamaagoowiziwaad ingiw niiyawen'enyag da-gabe-bimaadiziwaad dibishkoo a'aw Anishinaabe mewinzha ingodwaak miinawaa niishtana awashime gii-oditang gii-taso-biboonagizid. Weweni-go gashki'ewiziwaad weweni da-ganawenindizowaad da-ni-maajiikamigaanig i'iw aki.

[29] Da-wii-naadamaagoowiziwag da-ni-aabajitoosigwaa wenda-inigaa'igod a'aw Anishinaabe i'iw minikwewin naa anooj ani-aabajitood a'aw bemaadizid enigaa'igod. Ishke naniizaanendaagwadini naa wenda-mashkawaamagadini noongom eni-aabajitood a'aw bemaadizid.

[26] There are spirits that especially have compassion for our Anishinaabe children. I have always heard about those spirits coming to play with our children. Those are the spirits known as Little People in the Woods. I also offer the tobacco and the food to them to also watch over our new namesake.

[27] It is also here that I ask that my namesake be helped in their future, so that they do not bump into sicknesses that we cannot see. I also plan to ask that my namesakes be helped to eat the right foods that will keep them healthy. There are a lot of foods out there today that Anishinaabe eat that cause different illnesses such as diabetes, high blood pressure, and heart troubles.

[28] I also plan on asking that my namesakes be helped to live a good long life much like our Anishinaabe of the past who lived to be one hundred and twenty plus years in age. I ask that my namesakes are able to take good care of themselves in their future.

[29] I also ask that my namesakes be helped to stay away from using alcohol and drugs, which has done a lot of damage to us as Anishinaabe. What is being used today is dangerous and really powerful.

[30] Da-wii-naadamaagoowiziwan inow ogitiziiman da-ni-ganawenimigod a'aw niiyawen'enh. Gego da-wii-manezisiiwag gegoo. Miinawaa gaye odaa-wii-gikinoo'amaagoon inow ogitiziiman da-ni-manaajitood omaa eyaamagak omaa akiing biinish gaye inow owiiji-bimaadiziiman, miinawaa da-wenda-gikendang da-ni-manaajitood miinawaa da-ni-apiitendang a'aw Anishinaabe gaa-izhi-miinigoowizid enakamigizid ani-asemaaked. Miinawaa ninanaandonge a'aw niiyawen'enyag wenjida ani-abinoojiinyensiwiwaad da-ganawenimigowaad inow Manidoon megwaa nibaawaad.

[31] Giishpin a'aw bezhig ge-wiiyawen'enyikawind imaa ayaasig, awiya-go odaa-naabibiitaagoon da-ni-naabishkaagenid i'iw wiisiniwin imaa gaa-achigaadeg. Gomaapii dash waabamind iniw asemaan da-miinaa.

[32] Mii dash gaye omaa iko minwendamaan gashkapinaawaad inow asemaan waa-miinindwaa waa-wiiyawen'enyikawinjig. Ishke dash imaa bezhig ayaasig waa-wiiyawen'enyikawind, mii imaa da-ishkosed a'aw asemaa gaa-kashkapijigaazod. Mii dash imaa da-naadamaagoowiziwaad ingiw weniijaanisijig da-wanendanzigwaa da-miinaawaad inow gaa-ayaasinijin ge-wiiyawen'enyikawiminjin owapii gii-tanakamigizing.

[33] Ishke dash gaye ingiw nawaj igo eni-gichi-aya'aawijig wii-miinigoowiziwaad i'iw anishinaabewinikaazowin, mii eta-go iniw asemaan ge-miinaawaad iniw gaa-inendaagozinijin da-wiindaawasonid. Gaawiin memwech wiisiniwin odaa-atoosiin. Mii a'aw bezhig mindimooyenyiban gaa-izhi-gikinoo'amawid.

[34] Misawaa-go gichi-aya'aawid a'aw Anishinaabe booch igo da-miinigoowizid da-anishinaabewinikaazod. Ishke bezhig a'aw inini gii-niizhwaasimidana-ashi-naano-biboonagizi gii-miinag o'ow anishinaabewinikaazowin.

[30] I also ask those spirits to help the parents take care of my namesake. That they are not lacking and are not without anything. I also ask that the parents are able to teach my namesake to respect everything that is on this earth, to be respectful to other people, and to hold respect and high regard for the ceremonies we have been given as a people. I also ask the spirits that they watch over my namesake while he or she sleeps, especially as a baby.

[31] If one of those that has been selected as a namesake is not there, somebody can sit for them and accept the food on their behalf. When the parents see them at a later date, they can give that person some tobacco.

[32] This is where I like it when the parents make tobacco ties to give to the namesakes that they have selected. If one of the individuals that was selected as a namesake was not there, they will have one tobacco tie remaining as a visible reminder to be sure to give tobacco to the individual that was not there at the time of the ceremony.

[33] Also for those Anishinaabe that are older and in need of an Anishinaabe name, they only have to give tobacco to the person that has to give out names. It is not necessary to have food as a part of their offering. That is what one of the old ladies taught me.

[34] It does not matter what age an Anishinaabe is; it would be ideal that they have an Anishinaabe name. There was one elder that was seventy-five years old when I gave him his Anishinaabe name.

[35] Aanind a'aw Anishinaabe omisawendaan i'iw giizhaa asemaa da-miinind dabwaa-wiindaawasod, mii dash imaa besho asaad iniw asemaan nibaad. Mii imaa nanaandomaad iniw Manidoon da-bi-wiindamaagod ge-izhinikaazonid iniw abinoojiinyensan. Mii gaye niin ayaapii ezhichigeyaan. Aaningodinong gaawiin omaa gayat aanind a'aw Anishinaabe nimiinigosiin. Mii-go bijiinag dabwaa-maajitaang mooshkina'aad inow indoopwaaganan.

[36] Mii dash iko ayaapii ezhichigewaad ingiw weniijaanisijig iniw abinoojiinyensan, gegoo iko omiinaawaan iniw ge-wiiyawen'enyikawaawaajin maagizhaa gaye waabooyaanan, meshkwadooniganan, anooj igo gegoo. Mii iw epigaabawiwaad ingiw weniijaanisijig. Mii imaa besho da-achigaadenigiban i'iw wiisiniwin gaa-achigaadenig. Mii a'aw eni-gaagiigidod ge-ni-apagizondamawaapan iniw Manidoon gaye da-ondiniged dash a'aw abinoojiinyens da-naadamaagoowizid. Ani-giizhiitaang, mii dash ininamawindwaa ge-naabishkaagejig, mii dash iwidi ani-dagoshimoonagak enabiwaad ingiw Manidoog.

[37] Mii-ko a'aw Anishinaabe eni-wanendang iniw meshkwadooniganan da-miinaad iniw gaa-anoonaajin da-bi-ganoodamaagowaad, wenjida waasa wenjiinid. Ishke nebowa izhise ani-biinjibajiged awiya chi-inagindeg noongom i'iw waazakonenjiganaaboo.

[38] Aanind ingiw ge-wiiyawen'enyikawinjig odayaanaawaa iko maanaawaad owiiyawen'enyimiwaan. Maagizhaa gaye iniw dewe'igaansan, maagizhaa gaye miigwanan, maagizhaa gaye opwaaganan. Mii iniw Manidoon gaa-igowaad da-izhichigewaad. Mii dash i'iw odizhi'on a'aw ge-wiiyawen'enyikawind ezhi-wiinjigaadeg. Mii dash imaa wendiniged a'aw maanind i'iw odizhi'on, mii iw ge-ni-naadamaagod oniigaaniiming.

[35] Some Anishinaabe like to be given their tobacco ahead of time before they give a name, so they can put it next to their bed. That is where that person calls on those spirits to come and give them an Anishinaabe name to give to that child. That is also what I do every now and then. Sometimes some Anishinaabe will not give me tobacco ahead of time. They will not give me tobacco until the start of the ceremony at the time they fill my pipe.

[36] Some of the Anishinaabe that are doing this ceremony for their child will give an offering to those they have selected as namesakes by giving them maybe a blanket, maybe some money, or various items. This is additional offering they are putting for their child. Those items can be placed next to the food that has been put down for the ceremony. The one speaking for the ceremony can offer it up to the spirits as a source of additional support for the child. When the ceremony is done, the items can be passed out to those that are attending the ceremony. By doing that, those items will go to those spirits.

[37] Sometimes Anishinaabe will forget to give a money offering to the one asked to give a naming ceremony. It is important to give a money offering to the speaker especially if he traveled a great distance. It costs a lot nowadays with the cost of gasoline.

[38] Some of those that have been selected as namesakes have been told by the spirits what to give their namesake as a source of support in their future. Some of them give small drums like a hand drum, or maybe a feather, or even a pipe. The spirits have told these people to give that to their namesakes. That becomes the child's sacred item that will give them spiritual help in their future.

[39] Nebowa iko Anishinaabe owanendaan
anishinaabewinikaazod. Ishke dash mii i'iw ge-izhichigepan
endasing asemaan asaad odaa-wiindamawaan iniw Manidoon
ezhinikaazod. Mii dash gaawiin odaa-wanendanziin
ezhinikaazod.

[40] Ishke dash aanind wenendangig odizhinikaazowiniwaa
mii-go ge-izhi-aabajitoowaapan ezhinikaazonid bezhig iniw
owiiyawen'enyimiwaan. Ishke dash gaye aanind nimiinaag
da-oshki-anishinaabewinikaazowaad. Mii dash omaa ani-
gaagiizomagwaa ingiw Manidoog, gaawiin nizhiigwaakwananziin
gayat gaa-izhi-miinigoowizid da-izhinikaazod.

[41] Ishke dash enendaagozijig ingiw ge-wiiyawen'enyikawinjig
ge-izhichigewaad, mii-go apane ani-waabamaawaad, mii
imaa da-ni-naazikawaawaad da-mino-doodawaawaad
weweni da-bizindawaawaad iniw owiiyawen'enyimiwaan.
Ominwendaanaawaa ingiw abinoojiinyag gaye wiinawaa
mino-doodawindwaa. Ishke aanind ingiw niiyawen'enyag
zhooniyaansan nimiinaag waabamagwaa. Giishpin a'aw
abinoojiinh wani'aad iniw ogitiziiman, mii iniw bezhig iniw
ge-wiiyawen'enyijin ge-ni-ganawenimigojin.

[42] Daa-wenda-zanagad aana-wii-mino-doodawagwaa bebezhig
ingiw niiyawen'enyag i'iw akeyaa gaa-izhi-gikinoo'amaagooyang
da-doodawangwaa giiyawen'enyiminaanig, onzaam nebowa
indayaawaag. Ishke noongom awashime niiwaak indayaawaag
niiyawen'enyag.

[39] Many of our Anishinaabe people forget their Anishinaabe name. To help Anishinaabe remember their Anishinaabe name, they can tell the spirits their Anishinaabe name each time they offer their tobacco. And that will help them to not forget their Anishinaabe name.

[40] For those who have forgotten their Anishinaabe name, they can use an Anishinaabe name of one of their namesakes. And I also give some Anishinaabe new names. I ask for compassion from those spirits, saying I am not excluding the Anishinaabe name they were originally given.

[41] What the namesakes can do is approach their namesakes each time they see them to treat them good and listen to them carefully. Young children like to get attention and to be treated respectfully. For some of my namesakes I will give them money whenever I see them. Our teaching is that if a child should lose one of his parents, it is one of his namesakes that will take care of him from there on out.

[42] It would be difficult for me to do right by all my namesakes in the way that we were taught as Anishinaabe to do for our namesakes, because I have so many. Today I have over four hundred namesakes.

[43] Ishke gaawiin aapiji ayaasiin noongom a'aw Anishinaabe
eni-wiindaawasod. Ishke nebowa a'aw gidanishinaabeminaan
gaawiin nitaa-ojibwemosiin biinish gaye gaawiin ogikendanziin
aaniindi ge-ondinang awiya ani-wiindaawasod. Ishke awiya
ani-wiiyawen'enyikawind inow abinoojiinyan weweni bebezhig
owiikwajitoon da-mino-doodawaad. Ishke dash onzaam nebowa
niiyawen'enyag indayaawaag, aaniish naa booch da-wii-
ayaamowaad anishinaabewinikaazowaad, mii iw apane wenji-
nakodamaan anoonigooyaan da-wiindaawasoyaan.

[44] Ishke dash ayaapii nigaagiizomaag ingiw Manidoog, gaawiin
nibaapinendanziin gaa-izhi-ina'oonwewiziyang. Ishke gaawiin
geyaabi nebowa ayaasiiwag eni-wiindaawasojig. Apegish dash
a'aw Anishinaabe ani-ayaangwaamitood da-ni-gikendang i'iw
Ojibwemowin nebowa dash da-ayaawaad ge-miigiwejig iniw
anishinaabewinikaazowinan.

[45] Ishke aaningodinong niwanenimaag awenenag aawiwaad
ingiw niiyawen'enyag. Mii dash enagwaa iko, "Bi-naazikawishig
ingoji waabamiyeg baa-ayaayaan. Bi-wiindamawishig
ezhinikaazoyeg. Ishke omaa bi-wiindamawiyeg ezhinikaazoyeg,
mii dash igo ge-ikidoyaan, "Wa! Mii sa naa niiyawen'enh!"
Mii i'iw ge-naadamaagoyaan da-gikeniminagog. Onzaam
nebowa niiyawen'enyag indayaawaag. Gaawiin gakina
inga-minjimenimaasiig."

[46] Ishke dash mii imaa waabanjigaadeg ani-wanitooyang
eshkam i'iw akeyaa gaa-izhi-miinigoowiziyang. Nebowa
iko gii-ayaawag gaa-wiindaawasojig. Ishke dash noongom
eshkam ani-bangiiwagiziwag. Mii imaa waabanjigaadeg geget
ginishwanaaji'igonaan a'aw wayaabishkiiwed. Eshkam nebowa
a'aw Anishinaabe ani-bagijwebinang gaa-izhi-miinigoowiziyang
i'iw akeyaa da-ni-bimiwidooyang bimaadiziyang
anishinaabewiyang.

[43] Today there are very few that give Anishinaabe names. A lot of our Anishinaabe today are not able to speak our language and do not know where these Anishinaabe names come from that are given out. When someone is given a child as a namesake he should work at paying attention to each one of them. Even though I have too many namesakes, I still agree to do the ceremony and the naming, because I want our Anishinaabe to have an Anishinaabe name.

[44] Every so often I ask those spirits to have compassion for me and tell them that I am not being disrespectful to our teachings. Nowadays there are not many who give Anishinaabe names anymore. I hope that the Anishinaabe work hard at learning the Ojibwe language, so that there are many that can give Anishinaabe names.

[45] At times I forget who my namesakes are. I often say to them, "Come approach me whenever you see me, and let me know your Anishinaabe name. Once you tell me what your Anishinaabe name is, I would say, *Oh, yes! This is my namesake!* That is what will help me in knowing that you are my namesake. I have far too many namesakes. I could not possibly remember them all."

[46] This is where it shows that we have lost a lot of what we were given. There used to be plenty of people who gave Anishinaabe names. Nowadays there are a lesser number of people who give names. This is a visible sign on how distracting the white man has been for us. More and more of our Anishinaabe are dropping the way that we were given to live our lives as Anishinaabe.

[47] Ishke a'aw bezhig niiyawen'enh iniw onaabeman gaa-
izhichigenid, mii-go apane gii-miikinzomid, anooj gii-izhid.
Mii dash a'aw niiyawen'enh gaa-niibawitawid gii-wiindamawid
"Gego babaamitawaaken ekidod a'aw niwiijiiwaagan." Mii iw
nebowa ingiw Anishinaabeg gaa-izhichigewaad, gaawiin dash
geyaabi aapiji niwaabandanziin da-izhichiged i'iw akeyaa a'aw
Anishinaabe.

[48] Ishke dash awiya miinigoowizid odanishinaabewinikaazowin,
mii iniw weweni endoodawaajin biinjina eyaawaajin, iniw
ojichaagwan. Anishinaabewiwan iniw. Ishke dash oniigaaniiming
ge-ni-izhichigepan, nawaj da-ni-mino-doodawaad iniw
ojichaagwan, odaa-wii-gikendaan da-ni-anishinaabemod,
miinawaa da-ni-naazikang gaa-miinigoowizid a'aw Anishinaabe
ani-asemaaked, miinawaa endaso-giizhik asemaan da-asaad.

[49] Miinawaa weweni da-ni-naanaagadawendang, gego da-ni-
maji-inendanziin. Miinawaa gakina bebezhig anishinaabewiyang
apii gii-asigooyang omaa Manidoo odakiiming, gegoo-go gigii-
inendaagozimin da-izhichigeyang megwaa maa bibizhaagiiyang
omaa akiing. Mii iw ge-nandawaabandamang megwaa maa
ayaayang omaa akiing, da-ni-giizhiikamang idash. Mii dash
imaa ge-ni-naadamaagoyang zakab biinjina da-ni-izhi-ayaayang,
weweni ani-doodawang omaa biinjina bemiwinang.

[47] The husband of one of my namesakes would always tease me every time he saw me, saying different things. And his wife who was my namesake would always stand up for me and say, "Do not listen to what my husband says." This is what a lot of our Anishinaabe did, but I no longer see our Anishinaabe people doing that.

[48] When a person is given an Anishinaabe name, they are doing good to their spirit within. That spirit is Anishinaabe. To further nurture their spirit, they can learn the Ojibwe language, attend ceremonies, and put out their tobacco every day.

[49] He should also work at having a peaceful mind and not have negative thoughts. Also each one of us as Anishinaabe when we were put on this earth, we were put here for a reason. There is something we are to accomplish while we are on this earth. This is what each Anishinaabe has to find out what they are to do while they are here on earth and to complete it. This will help us to have peace within when we nurture our Anishinaabe spirit within.

[50] Ishke ezhi-apiitendaagwak i'iw anishinaabewinikaazowin da-ayaang a'aw Anishinaabe. Mii imaa apii da-ni-aabajichigaadenigiban giishpin gegoo ani-maazhi-izhiwebizid a'aw Anishinaabe maagizhaa gaye chi-aakozid. Mii imaa ani-apa'iwed ani-manidooked a'aw Anishinaabe nanaandomaad inow Manidoon da-naadamaagod mino-ayaawin da-miinigoowizid. Ishke dash owapii ani-asaad inow asemaan miinawaa wiisiniwin naa awegonen igo waa-ni-atood waa-ni-apigaabawid, mii inow ge-ni-ganoodamaagojin da-wenda-minwiinid da-ayaaminid i'iw anishinaabewinikaazowin ge-ni-aabajitoonid da-ni-ganoodamaagod miinawaa inow Manidoon oga-wenda-gikenimigoon awenen aawid.

[51] Miinawaa ani-aanjikiid a'aw Anishinaabe, mii gaye da-ni-aabajichigaadenig odizhinikaazowin. Mii dash gidinawemaaganinaanig iwidi eyaajig da-ayaamowaad odizhinikaazowin ge-aabajitoowaad da-anamikaagod iwidi ani-dagoshimoonod ezhaad a'aw Anishinaabe gaagwiinawaabaminaagozid omaa akiing.

[52] Mii-ko anooj inagwaa ingiw Anishinaabeg i'iwapii miinigoowiziwaad ge-izhinikaazowaad, gayat dabwaa-miinigoowiziwaad odanishinaabewinikaazowiniwaa, mii-ko ingiw Manidoog gaa-ikidowaad "Mii a'aw aya'aa iniw odasemaan." Mii dash omaa noongom da-wenda-gikenimigowaad iniw Manidoon awenen aawiwaad.

[50] It is important that an Anishinaabe have their Anishinaabe name. Their Anishinaabe name can be used when they are having a hard time, maybe a serious illness. They will be running to our Anishinaabe ceremonies with their tobacco for the spirits asking that they are given good health. At this time they give an offering of tobacco, food, and other items. The one speaking on their behalf will be much more efficient in having their Anishinaabe name to use and those spirits will definitely know who they are.

[51] Also when an Anishinaabe changes worlds, that is the time that his Anishinaabe name will be used. And our relatives over there in that other world will have an Anishinaabe name to use when he is no longer seen on earth.

[52] As I tease Anishinaabe that are in the process of getting their Anishinaabe name, I will tell them that the spirits will say that is whatchamacallit's tobacco. And then I tell them from here on out that the spirits will know who they are and have an Anishinaabe name as referred to them.

10 OSHKI-BIINDIGED A'AW ABINOOJIINYENS IMAA NIIMI'IDING

[1] Mii dash imaa wii-ni-dazhindamaan oshki-biindiganind a'aw abinoojiinyens imaa niimi'iding apii aabajichigaazod a'aw Manidoo-dewe'igan. Ashi-bezhig ingiw Manidoo-dewe'iganag niganawendamaagemin omaa Misi-zaaga'iganiing ezhi-wiinjigaadeg. When the parents see them at a later date they can give that person some tobacco.

[2] Ishke dash inow ogitiziiman a'aw abinoojiinyens ezhichigenid, mii inow asemaan miinawaa i'iw wiisiniwin baandigadoonid omaa apii baakishimind a'aw Manidoo-dewe'igan. Mii-go omaa miinawaa gaabige achigaazonid odasemaan a'aw abinoojiinyens. Mii dash iwidi da-oshki-dagoshimoononid miinawaa iwidi enabiwaad ingiw Manidoog. Ishke imaa gayat niizhing gii-inikaawan inow odasemaan gaa-atamawind a'aw abinoojiinyens iwapii gii-oshki-daangishkang i'iw aki miinawaa iwapii gii-miinind odizhinikaazowin.

[3] Geget minochige a'aw Anishinaabe gaabige asaad asemaan mino-doodawaad inow oniijaanisan noomaya igo gaa-inendaagwadinig gii-pi-dagoshimoononid. Geget ominwendaanaawaadog ingiw Manidoog gaabige ani-mikwenimindwaa. Mii imaa ge-onjikaamagadinig a'aw abinoojiinh da-naadamaagoowizid oniigaaniiming.

10 THE FIRST TIME A BABY IS BROUGHT INTO A CEREMONIAL DANCE

[1] I am going to talk about the first time a baby is brought into a dance where a ceremonial drum is being used. We take care of eleven ceremonial drums here on the Mille Lacs Reservation.

[2] What the baby's parents do is bring in tobacco and food when a ceremonial drum is uncovered to be used. Here the tobacco goes out right away for the baby again. The baby's tobacco newly arrives over there again where those spirits sit. Prior to this, the baby's tobacco went to those spirits on two different occasions, with the ceremony where the baby's feet were first placed on the earth and when the baby was given a name.

[3] It is good when an Anishinaabe puts out tobacco right away. They are doing well by their baby who just recently arrived. The spirits must be happy that they are being remembered right away. It is from here that the baby will be helped in his future.

[4] Mii dash omaa nising weweni doodawaawaad inow Manidoon weniijaanisijig inow abinoojiinyensan. Geget gii-shawendaagozi a'aw Anishinaabe gii-miinigoowizid o'ow akeyaa da-ni-naadamaagoowizinid inow oniijaanisan. Ishke dash i'iw wiisiniwin baandigadoowaad, mii imaa boozikinaaganing achigaadeg. Mii i'iw wiisiniwin inow oninjiin aayaabajitood zhakamoonindizod awiya imaa echigaadeg boozikinaaganing.

[5] Mii dash a'aw bezhig inow ogitiziiman eni-izhichigenid, akawe omaa ogizhibaashkawaan inow Manidoo-dewe'iganan, mii dash imaa asemaan asaad inow Gimishoomisinaanin asemaawinaaganing. Mii dash eshkosed a'aw asemaa, mii iwidi o-ininamawaad waa-kanoodamaagowaajin. Mii dash imaa gaye a'aw Oshkaabewis atood anaakan awasayi'ii desapabiwining iko wawenabiwaad ingiw niimi'iwewininiwag ningaabii'anong iwidi akeyaa.

[6] Mii dash i'iw wiisiniwin miinawaa minikwewin baandigadoowaad da-achigaadeg ogijayi'ii imaa anaakaning. Mii dash a'aw eni-gaagiigidod, mii iw ani-apagizondamawaad inow Manidoon wayaakaabiitawaanijin inow Gimishoomisinaanin inow asemaan naa wiisiniwin gaa-pi-biindigadoonid inow ogitiziiman a'aw abinoojiinyens.

[7] Mii dash imaa nanaandomindwaa ingiw Manidoog da-maamawinikeniwaad da-ni-ganawenimaawaad inow abinoojiinyensan weweni da-izhi-ayaanid oniigaaniiming, mino-ayaawin miinawaa mino-mamaajiiwin da-miinigoowizinid inow abinoojiinyensan. Miinawaa inow ogitiziiman da-wawiingeziwaad da-ganawenimaawaad inow oniijaanisensiwaan da-ni-manezisigwaa gegoo oniigaaniimiwaang, da-zhawendaagoziwaad gaye omaa bi-waabanda'iwewaad ezhi-apiitendamowaad gaa-izhi-miinigoowiziyang anishinaabewiyang.

[4] This is the third time the parents are doing good to the spirits on behalf of their baby. The spirits really showed compassion to their Anishinaabe when they were given these ceremonies from which the baby is helped. Food that is brought in is put in a bowl. It is finger food that is put into that bowl.

[5] This is what one of the parents does; he or she walks around the drum, and places the tobacco in the drum's tobacco dish. They will then hand the remaining tobacco to the person they have selected to talk on behalf of their baby. The *Oshkaabewis* places a mat on the other side of the bench where the singers sit on the west side of the drum.

[6] The food that they have brought in along with the drink is placed on top of that mat. Then the one that is doing the speaking sends the tobacco and the food brought in by the parents of the baby off to the spirits that sit around the ceremonial drum.

[7] The spirits are asked to put their hands together to help the child be given good health and movement. They also ask that the spirits help the parents be efficient in taking care of their child, and not be lacking anything in their future; they also ask that the parents be helped for showing their appreciation for what the spirits have given us as Anishinaabe.

[8] Mii dash imaa da-onjikaamagadinig da-zhawendaagoziwaad miinawaa weweni da-ganawenjigaazonid oniigaaniiming inow oniijaanisensiwaan. Weweni gaye odaa-wii-gikinoo'amawaawaan oniijaanisiwaan o'ow akeyaa gaa-inendaagozid Anishinaabe da-ni-bimiwidood i'iw obimaadiziwin.

[9] Mii-go imaa gaye ani-miigwechiwi'indwaa ingiw Manidoog weweni omaa gii-pi-dagoshimoonod a'aw abinoojiinyens. Geget chi-ina'oonwewizi a'aw Anishinaabe miinigoowizid oniijaanisan. Ishke dash mii imaa nanaandongeng ingiw Manidoog da-wiidookawindwaa ingiw weniijaanisijig da-wawiingeziwaad da-gikinoo'amawaawaad inow oniijaanisensiwaan i'iw akeyaa gaa-izhi-miinigoowiziyang anishinaabewiyang. Mii ingiw gidabinoojiinyiminaanig ge-ni-bimiwidoojig niigaan gaa-izhi-miinigoowiziyang anishinaabewiyang.

[10] Ishke niin omaa ani-gaagiigidoyaambaan, mii imaa da-gii-nanaandomagwaaban ingiw Manidoog da-naadamaagoowizinid inow ogitiziiman da-ni-ayaangwaamitoowaad da-gikinoo'amawaawaad inow oniijaanisensiwaan da-ni-mamanaajitoonid gakina omaa eyaamagak omaa akiing biinish gaye inow owiiji-bimaadiziiman miinawaa weweni da-bizindawaad naa weweni da-odaapinang egod inow ogitiziiman naa-go gaye inow gechi-aya'aawinijin nanaginigod owapii gegoo ani-maazhichiged.

[11] Mii-go gaye oga-wii-gikinoo'amawaawaan inow oniijaanisensiwaan zakab da-wii-izhi-ayaanid bizaan imaa da-nanaamadabinid aaniin igo apii ani-naazikaminid ani-manidooked a'aw Anishinaabe. Mii iw noongom wenitooyang. Mii iw nesidawinaagwak noongom, gaawiin a'aw Anishinaabe ogikinoo'amawaasiin inow oniijaanisan i'iw akeyaa gaa-izhi-gikinoo'amawaawaad mewinzha.

[8] It is from there they will be given compassion and also from which the baby will be well taken care of in their future. They will also be given help to teach their child the way that the spirits intended the Anishinaabe to live their life.

[9] It is also here that the spirits are being thanked for the safe arrival of this baby. It is quite the gift for Anishinaabe to be given a baby. It is here also that help is requested from the spirits to help the parents be efficient in teaching their child the ways that we as Anishinaabe were taught to live our lives by the spirits. It is our children who will carry on the teachings we were given as a people.

[10] If I were doing the talking at this particular time, it is here that I would have asked the spirits to help the parents to work hard at teaching their child to respect everything on this earth and also their fellow human beings, and also for the child to listen carefully and to accept what he is being told by his parents and elders when he or she is being scolded for their wrongdoings.

[11] That they also teach their child how to be calm within and to sit quietly as they attend ceremonies. That is what we are missing today. It is apparent today that the Anishinaabe are not teaching these things to their children as it was done years ago.

[12] A'aw bezhig akiwenziiyiban gaa-ni-gaagiigidod, ogii-tazhindaan ishpiming imaa ombinind mamaajigaadenid a'aw abinoojiinyens, mii imaa waabanda'iwed ezhi-aanoodizid wii-niimid. Ani-giizhiitaad ani-gaagiigidod, mii dash a'aw Oshkaabewis ani-maajiidood i'iw wiisiniwin, mii dash imaa ani-maada'ookiid da-ni-naabishkaagenid imaa eyaanijin. Weweni ani-gizhibaashkaamagadini i'iw wiisiniwin, weweni inikaamagadinig iwidi ingiw Manidoog wayaakaabiitawaajig inow Manidoo-dewe'iganan.

[12] One of the old men that spoke at this ceremony talked about when you lift a child up you can see their legs kicking, which shows how anxious they are to dance. When the talking is finished, the *Oshkaabewis* takes the bowl of food and passes it around to the people present to accept the food on behalf of the spirits. The food is passed around the circle of people attending and in turn it goes to the spirits that sit in a circle around the drum.

11 AADIZOOKENG

[1] Mii omaa wii-ni-wiindamaageyaan gaa-izhi-gikinoo'amaagooyaan ingiw aadizookaanag gii-tazhinjigaazowaad. Mii eta-go iko biboonagak apii eni-aadizooked awiya miinawaa azhigwa gaa-pangishimod a'aw giizis.

[2] Ishke dash gaye niwii-wiindamaage azhigwa oshki-bangishing a'aw goon, booch da-asemaakawaad a'aw Anishinaabe inow Manidoon omaa eyaanijin gooning. Mii a'aw Gaa-biboonike ezhi-wiinind a'aw Manidoo.

[3] Ishke dash azhigwa a'aw goon gii-ayaad, mii owapii eni-naazikawind netaa-aadizooked. Booch weweni da-doodawind, asemaan da-miinind, miinawaa gemaa waabooyaan da-miinind, miinawaa aniibiish ge-minikwed megwaa aadizooked mii gaye ge-miinind.

[4] Ishke booch da-biboonagak. Ishke giishpin eni-aadizooked awiya megwaa ayaasinig inow goonan, omakakiin oga-mikawaan imaa da-wiipemigod. Mii iw gaa-igooyaan.

[5] Ishke dash a'aw mindimooyenyiban gaa-nitaawigi'id, mii a'aw iko gaa-aadizookawid. Booch igo asemaan gii-miinag. Ishke dash gaye a'aw mindimooyenyiban gaa-izhid, "Wiikwajitoon da-goshkoziyan. Gego noonde-nibaaken dabwaa-giizhaajimag a'aw aadizookaan, ishke Manidoog ingiw endazhinjigaazojig omaa aadizookeng. Weweni bizindaman omaa enaajimoyaan, gegoo-go omaa gidaa-ina'oonwewiz ge-naadamaagoyan. Manidoog omaa endazhinjigaazojig omaa eni-aadizooked awiya. Gidaa-zhawenimigoog weweni bizindaman."

11 WINTER LEGENDS

[1] I am going to tell what I was told about our Winter Legends. It is only in the wintertime that these legends are told and it must be after the sun has gone down.

[2] I also want to tell that when the first snow falls a tobacco offering must be made to that spirit that exists within the snow. That spirit is known as *Gaa-biboonike* in our language.

[3] Once the snow has arrived, that is when you approach one who knows how to tell these legends. You must treat them respectfully and give them tobacco, and possibly even a blanket, and tea to drink while they are sharing their knowledge of the legends.

[4] It has to be winter. If someone were to go ahead and tell these legends without there being any snow on the ground, that person will find a frog sleeping with them. That is what I was told.

[5] It was the old lady that raised me that told me these Winter Legends. I always had to give her tobacco. This is what the old lady told me, "Please try to stay awake. Do not fall asleep before I finish telling a legend. These are spirits that are being talked about in these legends. If you listen carefully to what I am telling, you could be gifted with something from these legends that will help you, after all these are spirits that are talked about in these legends. They can gift you if you listen to these legends carefully."

[6] Ishke wiin a'aw Chi-mookomaan anooj inaajimod, gaawiin i'iw menidoowaadadinig odazhindanziin. Mii inow endazhindamaanin dibaajimowinan eyaangin a'aw Chi-mookomaan. Gaawiin omaa gegoo menidoowaadak onjikaamagasinini a'aw abinoojiinh ge-naadamaagod.

[7] Ishke dash a'aw Anishinaabe gakina gegoo ezhi-apiitendang, mii iko azhigwa gaa-aabita-biboong ingoji-go wapii maadaginzod a'aw Gichi-manidoo-giizis, mii a'aw mindimooyenyiban gii-azheyaajimaad iniw aadizookaanan gayat gaa-tazhimaajin. Mii imaa gii-wiindamawid wii-azhegiiwewinaad iniw Manidoon imaa aadizookaaning gaa-tadibaajimaajin gii-aadizooked weweni wii-azhenizha'waad gaa-onjikaanid.

[8] Mii dash iko apii gii-aadizooked a'aw mindimooyenyiban, mii imaa gii-aayaajimaad inow Wenabozhoyan. Nebowa aadizookaanag ayaawag eni-datazhinjigaazonid inow Wenabozhoyan. Ishke bezhig inow aadizookaanan gaa-wiindamawid, mii imaa gii-tazhimaad iniw gwiiwizensan. Omigiinaans gaa-izhi-wiinind. Miinawaa gaye aanind ingiw aadizookaanag gii-kinwaabiigiziwag. Niizho-dibik maagizhaa gaye niso-dibik gii-tazhitaa gii-kiizhaajimaad bezhig iniw aadizookaanan. Miinawaa nebowa imaa ayaamagad ani-gikinoo'amawind a'aw abinoojiinh i'iw gwayak da-ni-bimiwidood i'iw akeyaa izhi-bimaadizid.

[6] When the white man tells his stories, there is nothing that is spiritual that he talks about. I am speaking of the stories that the white man tells. There is nothing helpful on a spiritual level that can come from his stories that would benefit a child when hearing these stories.

[7] To show that the Anishinaabe has respect for everything, when it would be midwinter or around the first of January, that old lady would retell the legends that she had told me up until that point. It is then that she told me that she was returning those spirits from those legends that she had told, to send them back to where they originally were.

[8] When that old lady told those legends, one of those spirits she talked about quite often was *Wenabozho*. There are a lot of these legends that talk about *Wenabozho*. One of the legends that she told me talked about a little boy. His name was Scabby Boy. Some of the legends she told me were lengthy. Sometimes it took her two to three nights for her to complete one of these legends. These legends consisted of a lot of teachings that will help a child live a good life, the way we should live our life as Anishinaabe.

12 GII'IGOSHIMOWIN

[1] Mii iko ingiw Anishinaabeg mewinzha gaa-izhichigewaad, azhigwa gii-moonenimind a'aw gwiiwizens ani-oshki-ininiiwid, naa gaye a'aw ikwezens ani-ikwewid, mii iwidi bagwaj gii-izhiwinindwaa gii-o-gii'igoshimowaad ezhi-wiinjigaadeg. Mii iwidi wiigiwaam gii-ozhichigaadenig imaa bagwaj. Mii dash imaa gii-asind a'aw waa-kii'igoshimod maagizhaa ingo-dibik, gemaa gaye niizho-dibik, gemaa gaye niso-dibik miinawaa gemaa gaye niiwo-dibik gii-ayaad iwidi.

[2] Ishke dash megwaa iwidi gii-ayaawaad, gaawiin ogii-minikwesiinaawaa gegoo, biinish gaye gemaa gaawiin gii-wiisinisiiwag. Mii dash i'iw gaa-onji-izhichigewaad, mii imaa gii-waabanda'iwewaad ezhi-apiitendamowaad gaa-izhi-gikinoo'amaagooyang anishinaabewiyang. Dibishkoo imaa waabanda'iwewag ezhi-apiitenimaawaad iniw Manidoon imaa ani-mamoosigwaa da-gii-minikwewaapan naa gaye da-gii-wiisiniwaapan.

[3] Ishke dash mii imaa gaa-onjikaamagadinig gii-shawenimigowaad iniw Manidoon, mii dash imaa gaa-onjikaamagadinig gii-pi-naazikaagowaad iniw Manidoon gii-pi-wiindamaagowaad i'iw akeyaa ge-ni-naadamaagowaad oniigaaniimiwaang. Ishke mii imaa gaa-onjikaawaad ingiw Anishinaabeg gaa-wenda-manidoowaadizijig miinawaa gaa-nanaandawi'iwejig naa-go gaye gaa-chiisakiijig.

12 FASTING

[1] What Anishinaabe did as soon as they realized that a boy was becoming a young man and a girl was becoming a woman, they took them out into the woods to fast. A wigwam was built for them out in the woods. It was within there that they placed the one who was to fast for a night, maybe two nights, maybe three nights, or even four nights.

[2] While they were out there, they did not drink anything and possibly they did not even eat out there. The reason they did this was that they were showing their respect for what we were taught to do as Anishinaabe. It was as if they were showing their appreciation for the spirits by not taking anything to drink or to eat.

[3] It is from there that the spirits showed their compassion for them. It is from there that the spirits approached them and told them how they would help them in their future. That is where our Anishinaabe who were really gifted as healers, doctors, and wigwam shakers came from.

[4] Ishke ani-minikwesig awiya miinawaa ani-wiisinisig megwaa iwidi gii'igoshimod mii iwapii dibishkoo ani-wiindamawaad inow Manidoon, "Ishke mii i'iw waa-poonitooyaan, mii dash imaa aazhita inendamaan Manidoodog da-naadamawiyeg da-miizhiyeg wenjida ge-naadamaagoyaan niniigaaniiming."

[5] Mii dash dibishkoo eni-izhichiged a'aw Anishinaabe ani-atood i'iw wiisiniwin maagizhaa gaye imaa zagaswe'idid gemaa gaye ani-biindigadood endazhi-niimi'idiiked a'aw Anishinaabe. Mii imaa eni-gaagiigidod ani-wiindamaaged, "Ishke i'iw wiisiniwin a'aw gaa-pi-biindigadood da-gii-ashamoonsipan, awashime dash omaa enendang wii-pi-biindigadood ininamawaad inow Manidoon. Mii imaa ge-onjikaamagadinig da-ni-naadamaagod inow Manidoon."

[6] Mii-go gaye dibishkoo a'aw Anishinaabe bi-biindigadood inow maamandoogwaasonan imaa atood okosijiged imaa Anishinaabe endazhi-niimi'idiiked. Ishke a'aw gaa-kashkigwaasod anooj da-gii-paa-izhichigepan, awashime dash imaa enendang ginwenzh inendaagwadinig gii-nanaamadabid gii-kashkigwaadang i'iw waabooyaan waa-ininamawaad inow Manidoon. Mii gaye imaa wenjikaamagadinig a'aw Anishinaabe da-naadamawind.

[7] Mii-go gaye meshkwadooniganan asaad a'aw Anishinaabe. Geget chi-apiitendaagozi a'aw meshkwadoonigan. Gaawiin gegoo gidaa-gashkitoosiimin da-ni-izhichigeyang noongom ayaawaasiwang. Ishke dash imaa baandiganaad iniw meshkwadooniganan da-gii-aabaji'aapan, mii imaa awashime inendang wii-ininamawaad iniw Manidoon, mii imaa wendiniged a'aw Anishinaabe gaye ani-naadamaagoowizid.

[4] When a person does not drink and does not eat while they are fasting, it is as if they are telling the spirits during that time, "I am not going to eat or drink and in return I am hoping you all as spirits will help me and give me what will help me in my future."

[5] It is very similar to when Anishinaabe put down food maybe in a feast, or maybe a ceremonial dance. The one speaking for their offering says, "The food that so-and-so brought in could have been used to feed themselves and their family, but instead they thought to bring it in here and offer it up to the spirits. It is from there that they will be helped by the spirits."

[6] It is the same thing when Anishinaabe bring in handmade quilts as an offering for the bundle at a ceremonial dance. See the one that did the sewing could have been out doing whatever; instead they chose to sit long hours sewing the blanket that they are going to offer the spirits. It is also from there that the Anishinaabe get their help.

[7] The same also applies when Anishinaabe put money down as an offering. Money is held in high regard. Without money nowadays, we would not be able to do a lot of things. So when the money is brought in that could have been used, and instead that person chose to offer it up to the spirits, and it is from there that Anishinaabe also get help.

[8] Mii iw gaa-izhi-gikinoo'amaagoowiziyang anishinaabewiyang, gaawiin debinaak gidaa-doodawaasiwaanaanig ingiw Manidoog. Booch gegoo-go da-ininamawangwaa bagosenimangwaa aazhita dash da-naadamoonangwaa ingiw Manidoog. Gaawiin i'iw biinizikaa gidaa-inendanziimin da-naadamaagoowiziyang. Mii-go dibishkoo gii'igoshimod awiya gii-minikwesig miinawaa gii-wiisinisig. Mii iw epenimod da-onjikaamagadinig naadamaagoowizid a'aw Anishinaabe.

[9] Ishke mii i'iw noongom eshkam wenji-bangiiwagiziwaad ingiw Anishinaabeg nenaandawi'iwejig. Gaawiin geyaabi izhichigaanaasiiwag ingiw weshki-bimaadizijig da-gii'igoshimowaad. Ishke mii ingiw wenjida meshkawaadizijig miinawaa wewiingezijig nenaandawi'iwejig ingiw gaa-miinigoowizijig da-nanaandawi'iwewaad imaa apii gii-kii'igoshimowaad. Mii imaa apii gii-pi-naazikaagowaad iniw Manidoon imaa apii gii-kii'igoshimowaad. Mii imaa apii gii-pi-wiindamaagowaad inow Manidoon da-ni-nanaandawi'iwewaad oniigaaniimiwaang naa gaye mii i'iwapii gii-pi-odisigowaad inow Manidoon waa-naadamaagowaajin da-nanaandawi'aawaad iniw owiiji-anishinaabemiwaan.

[10] Nebowa ayaawag noongom biinizikaa nenaandawi'iwejig. Gaawiin o'ow akeyaa owapii gii-kii'igoshimowaad gii-miinigoowizisiiwag da-nanaandawi'iwewaad maagizhaa gaye gaawiin gii-kii'igoshimosiiwag gii-aya'aansiwiwaad. Nindaanawenimaag wiin ingiw biinizikaa dibishkoo nenaandawi'iwejig noongom.

[11] Ishke geget ochi-naadamaagon bagwaj imaa izhaad weshki-bimaadizid. Mii imaa ani-waabanda'igoowizid naa wenda-gikendang iniw Manidoon zhewenimigojin. Ishke noongom nebowa a'aw weshki-bimaadizid inigaawendam miinawaa aanawenindizo onji gii-o-gii'igoshimosig.

[8] We as Anishinaabe were taught not to do things half-heartedly, especially in our offerings when asking for help from the spirits. We have to have an offering for them as we express our desire of them to help us. We cannot just think that out of the clear blue that we will be helped. That also applies to someone who is fasting, that we make a sacrifice and go without anything to drink or eat. That is what the Anishinaabe rely on, that those spirits see those sacrifices, and it is from there that Anishinaabe get their help.

[9] That is the reason why we have so few Anishinaabe that are medicine men or traditional healers. We no longer do that for our young people by putting them out to fast as they did long ago. It is those that were given their powers through fasting that were especially powerful and efficient as medicine men. It was while they were fasting that the spirits approached them. It was at that time that they were told that the spirits would help them to do their doctoring in their future, and it was also at that time that they were approached by those particular spirits that were going to help them in doctoring their fellow Anishinaabe.

[10] There are many instant medicine men today. At the time of their fasting they were not given that ability to doctor, or maybe they did not even go out to fast when they were younger. I have no faith in the abilities of those that are doctoring today who did not get their powers from fasting.

[11] It is really a lot of help to that young person who goes out to fast. It is at that time that young people are shown and really know that the spirits have compassion for them. Not having experienced that, a lot of our Anishinaabe are depressed and have low self-esteem.

[12] Ishke bi-zhawenimigod inow Manidoon o'ow akeyaa, geget ochi-naadamaagon. Biinish gaye mii imaa apii ani-wiindamaagoowizid ge-ni-biminizha'ang imaa megwaa bibizhaagiid omaa akiing. Mii i'iw gaye geget wenda-naadamaagod oniigaaniiming.

[13] Ishke dash noongom giwaabandaamin enaadizid a'aw weshki-bimaadizid ani-gaagiiwozhitood inendaagwadinig ani-nishwanaajitood owiiyaw ani-aabajitood enigaa'igod a'aw Anishinaabe. Mii i'iw ge-onji-ayaangwaamitooyang da-bi-azhegiiwemagak da-gii'igoshimod a'aw gidooshki-bimaadiziiminaanig.

[14] Mii dash owapii a'aw oshki-inini gii'igoshimod, mii iw Makadeked ezhi-wiinjigaadeg. Ishke i'iwapii a'aw gwiiwizens ani-oshki-ininiiwid, maagizhaa gaye i'iwapii bakaanigondaagang ani-gaagiigidod. Mii owapii bagwaj da-ni-izhaapan.

[15] Ishke dash mii owapii ogitiziiman maagizhaa gaye iniw odedeyan ininamaagod imaa oninjiin gii-atood i'iw wiisiniwin naa iwedi bezhig akakanzhe gii-atood. Mii dash imaa ininamaagod iniw odedeyan a'aw oshki-inini. Giishpin mamood i'iw wiisiniwin gaawiin mashi inendanziin bagwaj da-izhaapan. Ishke dash a'aw mamood i'iw akakanzhe, mii dash imaa wiindamaaged wii-kii'igoshimod.

[16] Ishke dash dabwaa-maajitaad da-gii'igoshimod, mii imaa zinigobidood i'iw akakanzhe imaa odengwaang, da-makadewiingwed dash megwaa bagwaj imaa wii-ayaad. Mii iw wenji-izhi-wiinjigaadeg makadeked a'aw gwiiwizens. Miinawaa booch iniw asemaan da-ayaawaad a'aw oshki-inini da-baa-aabaji'aad megwaa imaa gii'igoshimod. Miinawaa giishpin opwaaganan ayaawaad, mii gaye inow ge-aabaji'aajin megwaa bagwaj imaa wii-ayaad.

[12] When the spirits come and take pity on the young person at the time of fasting, this is what helps them in their future. It is also at this time the young person is told what he or she is to pursue while on this earth. This is what really helps them in their future.

[13] Today we see how the young people are carrying their lives. They are wandering with no purpose or clear direction in their life and wasting their lives away by using alcohol and drugs that have been harmful to us as Anishinaabe. That is why we have to strive toward bringing back fasting for our young people.

[14] When a young man fasts it is called *Makadeked*. It is at the time that a boy is becoming a man; maybe it is at the time when a change in his voice is heard as he talks. It is then that he could go out in the woods to fast.

[15] It is at that time one of his parents, maybe his father extends out his hands: in one hand he has food and in the other hand he has ash from the fire. It is then that his father extends his hands to the young man. If the young man takes the food, it means that it is not his time to go out in the woods to fast. If the young man takes the ash, he is letting it be known that he is ready to fast.

[16] Before the young man goes out to fast, he takes the ash and rubs it all over his face so that his face is all black while he is out fasting. That is why fasting for a young boy is known as *Makadeked*. The young man must also have tobacco on him to use while he is out fasting. And if he has a pipe, he can also use it while he is out there fasting.

[17] Ishke dash wii-ni-wawiingezid a'aw Anishinaabe
miinawaa debinaak wii-ni-doodawaasig iniw Manidoon,
akawe imaa da-zagaswe'idim asemaan miinawaa
wiisiniwin da-ininamawindwaa ingiw Manidoog giizhaa
da-nanaandomindwaa weweni da-zhawenimaawaad miinawaa
weweni da-ganawenimaawaad inow weshki-bimaadizinijin
megwaa imaa gii'igoshimonid. Miinawaa mii owapii gaye
ge-ni-aabajichigaazod a'aw Anishinaabe menidoowaadizid
da-izhiwinigod imaa bagwaj waa-kii'igoshimod. Mii inow ge-ni-
ganawenimigojin gaye megwaa imaa ayaad bagwaj ayaapii da-ni-
dibaabamigod gaye.

[18] Bebakaan igo gii-izhi-waawiindamawaawag ge-izhichigeng
i'iwapii bagwaj izhiwinaawaad inow weshki-bimaadizinijin.
Aanind ingiw ishpiming imaa mitigog odoozhitamawaawaan
da-nanaamadabinid inow waa-kii'igoshimonijin. Aanind gaye
mii-go imaa jiigayi'ii imaa mitigong gii-wawenabi'indwaa.
Wiigiwaam aanind ogii-ozhitamawaawaan igaye imaa biindig gii-
nanaamadabinid waa-kii'igoshimonijin. Ishke dash gaye aanind
azhigwa gaa-ni-giizhiitaawaad gii-kii'igoshimowaad mii imaa
madoodiswaning gii-piindiganindwaa gaye.

[19] Ishke dash a'aw ikwezens owapii ani-moonenimind ani-
ikwewid, mii owapii bagwaj ezhiwinind imaa wiigiwaaming
da-ayaad. Mii dash i'iw bakaaniged a'aw ikwezens ezhi-
wiinjigaadeg. Ishke dash megwaa iwidi gii-ayaad iwidi
wiigiwaaming, maagizhaa gaye azhigwa gaa-ni-giizhiitaad gii-
kii'igoshimod, mii iniw mindimooyenyan gii-gikinoo'amaagod
iw akeyaa ge-ni-izhi-bimiwidood bimaadizid i'iw ani-ikwewid
oniigaaniiming. Ishke mii iwapii wenda-mashkawaadizid ani-
ikwewid a'aw ikwezens. Ishke i'iw bezhig gikinoonowin megwaa
ani-bimisemagadinig, mii i'iw wenjida da-ni-ganawaabandang
eni-izhichiged.

[17] If the Anishinaabe want to be efficient and not do things half-heartedly to the spirits, a feast is held first where tobacco and food is offered to the spirits ahead of time, asking that they show compassion and watch over the young man that is about to go out and fast. It is also at that time that an Anishinaabe that is gifted maybe as a medicine man takes the young man out into the woods to do his fasting. It is also that same Anishinaabe that will watch over as he is fasting and check on him periodically.

[18] There are little differences in the way people are taught on what is to be done when they take a young man out into the woods to fast. Some were taught to make a platform up in a tree where the young man can sit as he fasts. Some were also told to sit by a tree as they fasted. There was also some who made a wigwam for the young man to sit in as he fasts. As some finished their fasting they were taken into a sweat lodge.

[19] When it is realized that a young girl is becoming a woman, it is then that she is taken out into the woods to stay in a wigwam. This is why it is known as *Bakaaniged,* because the young girl is removed from their home to a separate dwelling when she fasts. While the young girl is in the wigwam, or maybe after she has finished fasting, the old ladies would come in and cover the teachings that are important for her to remember as she goes on to be a woman. The time when a young girl is becoming a woman is the most powerful stage of her life. Throughout the year after the young woman has to be especially careful in what she does.

[20] Ishke i'iw gigii-miinigonaanig ingiw Manidoog
anishinaabewiyang ge-inanjigeyang, mii i'iw manoomin, biinish
gaye ingiw giigoonyag, biinish gaye ingiw anooj awesiinyag,
waawaashkeshiwag, waaboozoog, biinish gaye bagwaj
mayaajiiging. Gaawiin a'aw oshkiniigikwe odaa-michi-mamoosiin
i'iw gaa-miinigoowiziyang ge-inanjigeyang. Akawe bezhig i'iw
gikinoonowin da-baabii'o.

[21] Ishke megwaa ani-bimi-ayaamagadinig i'iw gikinoonowin
owapii gaa-pakaaniged, wii-tazhiikang maagizhaa gaye wii-
miijid gaa-miinigoowiziyang ge-inanjigeyang, akawe a'aw asemaa
da-achigaazo miinawaa da-zhakamoonind i'iw mesawendang
gaa-miinigoowiziyang da-miijiyang. Ishke dash mii eta-go apii
i'iw niiwing ininamawind a'aw emikwaanens imaa wiisiniwin
gii-achigaadeg. Mii dash azhigwa niiwing gaa-ininamawind i'iw
emikwaanens, mii dash iwapii zhakamoonind a'aw oshkiniigikwe.
Mii dash i'iw bijiinag da-ni-dazhiikangiban da-ni-maamiijipan
imaa gaa-shakamoonind.

[22] Mii iw akeyaa gaa-izhi-gikinoo'amaagoowiziyaang omaa
Aazhoomog naa-go gaye Minisinaakwaang. Mii eta-go apii
niiwing ininamawind awiya owapii megwaa gii-pimisemagadinig
i'iw gikinoonowin owapii gaa-kii'igoshimod a'aw oshkiniigikwe
gii-pakaaniged. Ishke dash ingiw gaa-wanitaasojig gaa-
wani'aajig iniw besho enawemaawaajin, mii eta-go aabiding
ininamawindwaa i'iw emikwaanens ani-zhakamoonindwaa gaa-
izhi-miinigoowiziyang da-inanjigeyang anishinaabewiyang.

[20] The spirits gave us food to eat as Anishinaabe, such as the wild rice, the fish, and the wild animals like the deer, rabbits, and the plants and berries that grow in the wild. The young woman cannot just go out and pick or harvest those foods that we were given to eat. She will have to wait a year before she can do that.

[21] During that year following her fast, if she is going to handle or eat those food that we have been given, tobacco has to be put down first and then she has to be spoon-fed that particular food that we were given by the spirits to eat. This is the only time the spoon of food is offered to her four times. When the food is offered to her on the fourth time, that is when the young girl is spoon-fed. It is then that she is able to handle and eat that particular food that she had been spoon-fed.

[22] This is the way that we were taught in the Lake Lena and East Lake districts of the Mille Lacs Reservation. This is the only time that the spoon is offered four times to the young woman who has fasted within the last year. For those who are grieving and have lost a relative close to them, the spoon is only offered up to them one time, as they are being spoon-fed the various foods that we were given to eat as Anishinaabe.

[23] Gii-kina'amawaawag ingiw oshkiniigikweg megwaa bimisemagadinig i'iw gikinoonowin apii gaa-pakaanigewaad, gaawiin odaa-dazhiikawaasiwaawaan iniw abinoojiinyan bebiiwizhiinyiwinijin. Miinawaa gii-kina'amawaawag, gaawiin daa-bagizosiiwag imaa ziibiing miinawaa zaaga'iganiing. Gaawiin gaye odaa-daanginanziinaawaa imaa bagwaj mayaajiiging wawaaj igo inow aniibiishan, miinawaa gaawiin mitigoon odaa-akwaandawaanaasiwaawaan. Odaa-banaajitoonaawaa imaa mayaajiiging imaa bagwaj, mii iw wenjida mashkawaadiziwaad ingiw oshkiniigikweg. Miinawaa ogii-gikinoo'amaagowaan iniw mindimooyenyan ingiw oshkiniigikweg, gaawiin daa-baazhijidakokiisiiwag imaa atemagadinig ininiwag miinawaa abinoojiinyag obiizikaaganiwaan.

[24] Gaawiin imaa besho daa-ni-izhaasiiwag atemagadinig iniw Manidoo-aabajichiganan wenjida opwaaganan. Ishke izhi-mashkawaadiziwaad ingiw ikwewag, mii-go imaa ani-banaajitoowaapan iniw Manidoo-aabajichiganan, gaawiin geyaabi da-ni-mashkawaadasininiwan iniw. Nimikwendaan gii-waabamagwaa ingiw mindimooyenyag, mii imaa dabazhish gii-minjiminamowaad iniw ogoodaasiwaan gegoo dash imaa ishpiming da-ni-inagoodesininig ogoodaasiwaan wenjida besho ani-ayaawaad iniw Manidoo-aabajichiganan etemagadinig.

[25] Ingii-pi-waabandaan iko gaye a'aw na'aanganikwe gaa-pi-wiij'ayaawiyangid, mii dash imaa ayaapii bekaanadinig onaagan, emikwaanens, naa onaagaans gii-aabajitood owapii gii-izhiwebizid ingiw ikwewag ezhiwebiziwaad. Mii-go gaye eni-izhichigewaad bezhigwan iniw onaagan, emikwaanens, naa onaagaans ani-aabajitoowaad megwaa ani-bimisemagadinig i'iw gikinoonowin owapii gaa-pakaanigewaad.

[23] During that year after the young woman had fasted she was forbidden to touch small children or infants. She was also forbidden from swimming in the rivers and the lakes. They were also told not to touch those things that grow out in the wild, even the leaves of plants, and they were also told not to climb the trees. That could affect the growth of those plants that grow in the wild, since this is the most powerful time in the young woman's life. The old ladies also taught these young women not to step over clothing that belong to men or small children.

[24] They were also not to go near sacred items, especially pipes. These young women were so powerful at this time they were told that they could nullify the power that exists in our sacred items; they will no longer have the power they had. I remember seeing those old ladies, they would reach down and pull their dresses in so that their dresses would not hang over anything, especially when they would go near any sacred items that were placed on the floor.

[25] When one of our in-laws used to stay with us, I saw that she used a different plate, spoon, and cup during that time of the month women have their menstrual cycles. The young women also did the same thing during that year following their fasting, by only using a different plate, spoon, and cup.

[26] Nigii-pi-noondawaag ingiw ikwewag ani-dazhindamowaad, gaawiin odaa-naazikanziinaawaa endazhi-manidoo-niimi'idiikeng miinawaa zagaswe'idid a'aw Anishinaabe, miinawaa midewi'iweng megwaa ani-izhiwebizid a'aw ikwe iko izhiwebiziwaad endaso-giizis. Gaawiin wiikaa nibi-noondanziin iw akeyaa da-ni-izhi-gikinoo'amaaged a'aw Anishinaabe. Mii ganabaj i'iw wenjikaamagak iwidi Bwaan-akiing, mii iw akeyaa izhi-gikinoo'amawindwaa ingiw Bwaanikweg. Gaawiin wiikaa nibi-noondawaasiig ingiw gechi-aya'aawijig da-gii-izhi-gikinoo'amawaawaad inow ikwewan.

[27] Mii a'aw nizigosiban Amikogaabawiikweban gaa-gikinoo'amawid a'aw isa Anishinaabekwe ezhichiged ani-bakaaniged miinawaa gaa-izhi-gikinoo'amawind. Ishke a'aw mindimooyenyiban nigii-wiindamaag azhigwa gaa-ni-giizhiitaad gii-pakaaniged iwidi wiigiwaaming gii-ayaad, mii dash i'iwapii gii-pi-naazikang gaa-taawaad, mii imaa giizhikaandagoon gii-achigaazonid da-ni-dakokaanaad megwaa gii-naazikang imaa endaawaad.

[28] Mii-ko iwapii gii-paa-gikinoo'amaageyaan a'aw Anishinaabe gaa-izhi-miinigoowizid niizh dash ingiw mindimooyenyag gii-ayaawag imaa a'aw Amikogaabawiikweban naa-go gaye Gaagebiikwe. Mii ongow gaa-naadamawijig gii-tazhindamaan ani-bakaaniged a'aw ikwe. Mii dash imaa wendinamaan ingiw mindimooyenyag wezhibii'amaan imaa ezhichiged a'aw ikwe bakaaniged.

[26] I would hear women saying that they should not go to our ceremonial dances, feasts, and the Midewiwin lodge during their monthly menstrual cycle. I have never heard this as part of Anishinaabe teachings. I believe these teachings come from Lakota/Dakota country. That is the teaching that Lakota/Dakota women are taught. I have never heard our elders from the past teach that to our women.

[27] My late aunt Julie Shingobe was the one who taught me what a young woman was to do when she fasted and what she was also taught during that time. That old lady told me when she finished fasting and was approaching their home, cedar was placed on the ground for her to step on as she walked up to the house.

[28] When we went out and about giving presentations on Anishinaabe teachings, there were two of the old ladies that were present at that time, Julie Shingobe and Misko Binayshi. They were the ones that helped me as I covered the fasting that young women went through. It is from them that I got the information that I am writing down about fasting.

13 OSHKI-NITAAGED A'AW ABINOOJIINH

[1] Geget a'aw Anishinaabe omanaajitoon gakina gegoo wenjida i'iw gaa-miinigoowiziyang ge-inanjigeyang anishinaabewiyang. Ishke ingiw awesiinyag mii ingiw nitam gaa-nakodangig wii-naadamawaawaad inow Anishinaaben ishkweyaang gaa-ayaanijin i'iwapii gii-moonenimind a'aw Anishinaabe ezhi-gidimaagizid i'iw bimaadiziwin. Mii owapii a'aw Niigaani-manidoo gii-pi-azhegiiwed gii-moonenimaad ezhi-gidimaagizinid iniw odanishinaabeman. Mii dash gii-nandwewemaad iniw Manidoon da-bi-naadamawind a'aw Anishinaabe. Mii dash nitam ingiw awesiinyag gaa-pi-zaagewejig gii-pi-waakaabiitawaawaad iniw Niigaani-manidoon. Mii dash iwapii gii-nakodamowaad wii-naadamawaawaad iniw Anishinaaben miinawaa gii-nakodamowaad ge-ondanjiged a'aw Anishinaabe iniw awesiinyan.

[2] Mii gaye ingiw akiwenziiyibaneg gaa-inaajimowaad iwapii a'aw Niigaani-manidoo gii-nandwewemaad iniw Manidoon da-bi-naadamawind a'aw Anishinaabe, mii a'aw gaa-pi-zaagewed a'aw gimishoomisinaan. Geget gii-mindido. Mii ingiw Anishinaabeg imaa gaa-ayaajig i'iwapii ogii-noondawaawaan ani-bimi-ayaanid iwidi giiwedinong ani-ditibishing a'aw gimishoomisinaan. Mii dash owapii iniw zaaga'iganiin miinawaa ziibiwan gii-ozhichigaadeg da-onda'ibiid a'aw Anishinaabe. Mii dash owapii wii-gitigaazod a'aw giigoonh miinawaa i'iw manoomin. Mii dash i'iw wenji-manaajitood gaa-miinigoowizid a'aw Anishinaabe da-inanjiged, ingiw Manidoog gigii-miinigonaanig miinawaa gii-shawenimaawaad odanishinaabemiwaan. Ishke dash mii iw wenji-asemaaked naa zagaswe'idid oshki-nitaaged awiya.

13 A CHILD'S FIRST KILL

[1] The Anishinaabe treat everything respectfully, especially the foods we were given to eat as Anishinaabe. It was the animals that first came forward and agreed to help the Anishinaabe when they realized how pitiful the Anishinaabe were. It was at that time that the Creator realized how pitiful his Anishinaabe were and came back. It was then that he called on the spirits to come help the Anishinaabe. It was the animals that first appeared and sat around the Creator. It was at that time that they agreed to help the Anishinaabe and be a source of food for the Anishinaabe.

[2] The old men also said that while the Creator was there calling on the spirits to help the people, a large spirit also appeared. That spirit was really big. The Anishinaabe that were there at that time heard that spirit rolling in the north. It was at that time that the lakes and the rivers were created, giving the Anishinaabe a place to get their water. It was at that time that the fish were planted along with the wild rice. That is why the Anishinaabe treat those foods respectfully, because it was a gift to us from those spirits and a reflection of their compassion for us. So this is why the Anishinaabe does a tobacco and food offering at the time a young person kills his first animal or deer, or catches their first fish.

[3] Ishke dash gii-kwiiwizensiwiyaan, mii a'aw wayeshkad a'aw giigoonh gaa-tebibinag gaa-agwaawebinag, mii a'aw namebin ezhi-wiinind. Azhigwa gaa-pi-giiweyaan, mii a'aw mindimooyenyiban gaa-nitaawigi'id mii iw gaabige gii-ozhiitaad gii-chiibaakwed gii-sagaswe'idiyaang weweni gii-toodawaawaad iniw giigoonyan gaa-oshki-debibinimagin.

[4] Akawe sa wiin igo ogii-nandomaawaan inow nizhishenyibanen, mii inow gaa-nitaa-wewebanaabiinijin. Mii dash gaa-ikidowaad, "Mii imaa ge-ondinaman da-wenda-nitaa-wewebanaabiiyan giniigaaniiming miinawaa apane da-wenda-waanaji'adwaa giigoonyag."

[5] Mii dash a'aw akiwenziiyiban gii-mooshkina'aad iniw odoopwaaganan, gaa-ni-giizhiitaad ani-naabishkaaged iniw asemaan, mii dash iwidi gii-apagizomaad iniw asemaan miinawaa i'iw wiisiniwin enabiwaad ingiw Manidoog gii-miigwechiwitaagozid gii-miinigoowiziyang anishinaabewiyang a'aw giigoonh da-amwang miinawaa da-ni-naadamaagoowiziyaan gaye niin da-wenda-nitaa-wewebanaabiiyaan niniigaaniiming.

[6] Mii dash gaye gaa-izhichigewaad i'iw wayeshkad gii-nitooyaan gegoo. Mii a'aw akiwenziiyiban mitigwaabiin naa bikwak nigii-ozhitamaag da-aabaji'ag da-giiwoseyaan. Mii dash a'aw wayeshkad gaa-nisag mii a'aw bineshiinh. Mii-go dibishkoo gaa-izhichigewaad. Weweni asemaa miinawaa wiisiniwin gii-atoowaad miinawaa gii-nandomaawaad netaa-giiwosenijin. Mii-go imaa miinawaa weweni gii-toodawindwaa ingiw Manidoog miinawaa a'aw bineshiinh gaa-nisag.

[3] When I was a young boy, the first fish that I caught was a sucker. When I came home the old lady that raised me started to do her cooking so that we could feast as a way to treat the fish that I first caught respectfully.

[4] Before we feasted they called on an uncle of mine who they considered to be a good fisherman. It was then that I was told, "It is from there that you will get your ability to be a good fisherman and that you will never be lacking for fish."

[5] That old man filled his pipe; once he had smoked it he then offered the tobacco and food to where all the spirits sit, thanking them for giving us as Anishinaabe the fish to eat and asking for me to be helped to be an especially good fisherman in my future.

[6] They did the very same thing when I had my first kill. The old man made me a bow and arrow to use when I hunted. The first thing that I had killed was a bird. They did the very same thing. They put out tobacco and food and invited a person who was considered a good hunter to the feast. It was there that the spirits were treated respectfully and also the bird that I killed.

[7] Ishke a'aw gwiiwizens owapii oshki-nisaad iniw waawaashkeshiwan, mii gaye imaa apii a'aw asemaa naa wiisiniwin gii-achigaadeg. Mii i'iw aanind a'aw Anishinaabe ezhichiged, mii imaa okaakiganaang a'aw waawaashkeshi mii imaa wendinigaadeg i'iw wiiyaas eshangeng iwapii zagaswe'idid. Mii i'iw aanind gaye a'aw Anishinaabe ezhichiged, mii a'aw gwiiwizens gaa-nitaaged mii-go ezhi-miigiwed gakina i'iw waawaashkeshiwi-wiiyaas ashamaad iniw gechi-aya'aawinijin.

[8] Ishke dash gaye aanind a'aw Anishinaabe gaa-izhi-gikinoo'amawind i'iwapii oshki-nisaad iniw waawaashkeshiwan, mii-go imaa gaabige zhakamoonind a'aw gwiiwizens i'iw wiiyaas imaa gaa-ondinigaadenig o'ow ode'ing a'aw waawaashkeshi.

[7] When a young man kills his first deer, a tobacco and food offering is also made. What some of our Anishinaabe do, they get the meat from the chest of the deer and that is the meat that is offered up in the feast. What some Anishinaabe also do is that the young man who just killed his first deer gives all the deer meat away to the elders.

[8] What some of our Anishinaabe also do is soon after a young man kills his first deer, a piece of the meat is cut from the heart of that deer and is given to the young man to eat.

14 GIKINOO'AMAWIND MIINAWAA NANAGININD A'AW ABINOOJIINH

[1] Booch da-gikinoo'amawind a'aw abinoojiinh gaa-
ina'oonwewizid a'aw Anishinaabe. Ishke mii ingiw
giniigaaniiminaang ingiw ebinoojiinyiwijig noongom ge-ni-
bimiwidoojig gaa-izhi-miinigoowiziyang anishinaabewiyang.
Ishke a'aw abinoojiinh mii-go gaye wiin ezhichiged ani-
gikinawaabamaad eni-waabandang eni-izhichigenid iniw
ogitiziiman.

[2] Ishke noongom weniijaanisijig, mii iw ge-izhichigewaapan
endaso-giizhik iniw odasemaawaan da-asaawaapan. Agwajiing
odaa-asaawaan iniw odasemaawaan ani-bimi-ayaanid iniw
Binesiwan. Odaa-biindaakoodoonaawaa waa-mamoowaad bagwaj
waa-aabajitoowaad. Odaa-naazikaanaawaa a'aw Anishinaabe
okwi'idid ani-biindaakoojiged anooj inakamigizid. Weweni
daa-ozhiitaawag da-dazhiikamowaad waa-pagijigewaad
ani-naazikamowaad ani-manidooked a'aw Anishinaabe. Daa-
anishinaabemotaadiwag imaa endaawaad. Ishke mii a'aw
abinoojiinh ge-waabandang, mii dash gaye wiin ge-ni-izhichiged
ge-ni-inaadizid oniigaaniiming.

[3] Ishke ginwenzh igo nibi-naadamawaa ani-ganoodamawag
iniw odasemaan a'aw Anishinaabe ani-biindaakoojiged.
Ishke dash ingiw aanind gaa-naadamawagig ishkweyaang,
azhigwa gaa-ishkwaa-ayaawaad niwenda-minwendaan
waabandamaan oniijaanisiwaan ani-bimiwidoonid iniw
ogitiziimiwaan gaa-izhichigenid gii-pimaadizinid. Ishke mii
imaa wenjida ani-waabanjigaadenig gaa-izhi-wawiingezinid
ogitiziimiwaabanen weweni gii-gikinoo'amaagowaad geyaabi ani-
gikinawaabiwaad ani-bimiwidoowaad iniw ogitiziimiwaabanen
gaa-wenda-apiitendaminid.

14 TEACHING AND DISCIPLINING OUR CHILDREN

[1] We have to teach our children what we have been given as Anishinaabe. Our children are the ones who will be carrying on the teachings we have been given as Anishinaabe into the future. A child learns from observing his or her parents and in turn does the same.

[2] What our parents can do on a daily basis is offer up their tobacco. They can put their tobacco outside as they hear the Thunder-beings going by. They can offer up their tobacco to the plants in the wild that they plan to use. They can also attend the ceremonies where the Anishinaabe are offering up their tobacco. They can prepare for these ceremonies by putting their offerings together in a good way that they plan to use in these ceremonies. They can also use the Ojibwe language as they speak to one another in the home. This is what the young child will observe and will also continue to live his or her life in the same manner.

[3] I have been speaking for the Anishinaabe's tobacco for a good length of time. I really like seeing that some of the Anishinaabe I have helped in this way, that once they have passed on their children continue to carry on in the same way as their parents did. It really shows how efficient the parents were in teaching their children that they still continue to carry on the same practices that their parents valued.

[4] Daa-nanaginaa a'aw abinoojiinh. Ishke a'aw mindimooyenyiban gaa-nitaawigi'id mii iw gaa-ikidod, "Gaawiin gidinigaa'aasiin a'aw abinoojiinh nanaginad. Gimino-doodawaa." Ishke noongom niwaabamaag ingiw abinoojiinyag azhigwa ani-baakishimind a'aw Manidoo-dewe'igan ani-aabajichigaazod imaa niimi'iding, mii imaa gakina ingoji babaamibatoowaad imaa abinoojiinyag endanakamigak. Mii-ko gaa-igooyaan gii-kwiiwizensiwiyaan gii-wiiji'iweyaan gii-izhaayaan imaa endazhi-niimi'iding, "Bizaan omaa nanaamadabin. Mii eta-go ge-onji-bazigwiiyamban maagizhaa gaye da-niimiyamban gemaa gaye waakaa'igaansing da-izhaayamban."

[5] Ishke nigii-igoo "Giishpin babaamibatooyan omaa baakishing a'aw gimishoomisinaan bangishinan, gidaa-wenda-wiisagishin." Mii imaa gikinoo'amawind a'aw abinoojiinh da-apiitenimaad gimishoomisinaanin, aaniish naa mii iw iwidi gaa-onjikaanid iniw Manidoon gii-miinaanid iniw Anishinaaben da-apenimonid.

[6] Ishke dash gaye eko-maajaa'iweyaan, mii imaa noongom wenda-ombiigwewetoowaad abinoojiinyag babaamibatoowaad anooj izhichigewaad. Ishke mewinzha gaawiin ingiw abinoojiinyag gii-pagidinaasiiwag imaa da-bi-izhaawaad endazhi-maajaa'iweng. Ishke a'aw eni-gaagiigidod ani-maajaa'iwed, ishke imaa gegoo ani-noondang ombiigwewetoonid awiya, mii-go izhi-waniba'igod waa-ikidod.

[7] Ishke dash i'iw enendamaan noongom waabandamaan ingiw abinoojiinyag ezhichigewaad, mii-go imaa ani-naniizaanendamaan dibishkoo ani-naanaagadawendamaan aaniin ge-ni-inaadiziwaad oniigaaniimiwaang ingiw abinoojiinyag noongom. Ishke mii imaa wenjida da-ni-apiitendamawaawaapan iniw Manidoo-dewe'iganan, miinawaa weweni da-doodawaawaad inow gaa-ishkwaa-ayaanijin azhigwa waa-maajaanijin da-ni-aanjikiinid. Ishke ani-gichi-aya'aawiwaad, gaawiin gegoo oga-ni-apiitendanziinaawaa, mii dash geget da-nishwanaadizid a'aw Anishinaabe.

[4] A child should be disciplined. The old lady that raised me had said, "You are not doing a child harm when you discipline him or her. You are doing good to the child." I see that when we have our ceremonial dances and the drum is laid out to be used, the children are running all over the place in the dance hall. When I went along with those old people to the ceremonial dances as a young boy I was told, "Sit quietly. The only reason you need to get up is to go to the bathroom or to dance."

[5] I was also told, "If you were to run around while the ceremonial drum is being used, if you should fall you will hurt yourself badly." This is where a young child is taught to have respect for a ceremonial drum, after all the drum came from the spirits and was given to us as Anishinaabe to depend on for support.

[6] Ever since I started doing funerals, I noticed that especially nowadays, a lot of our children are making a lot of noise running around at the funeral site. A long time ago children were not allowed to be present at these funerals. When the one who is talking at the funeral hears some noise he will tend to forget what to talk about.

[7] When I see what our children are doing today I begin to be fearful as I think on how these children will conduct themselves in the future. They should especially have respect for the ceremonial drum when it is laid out and should be especially respectful to the spirit of the deceased who is about to leave and change worlds. What is scary about it all is to realize that when these young people get older, they will not have respect for anything, and this is when Anishinaabe will go downhill as a people.

15 GE-IZHI-GIKINOO'AMAWINDIBAN A'AW ABINOOJIINH

[1] Gego inigaa'aaken giday. Manidoowaadizi gaye a'aw animosh. Gakina gegoo-go manidoowaadad omaa akiing eyaamagak.

[2] Gego wanishkwemaaken megwaa mawadisidiwaad ingiw nawaj gechi-aya'aawijig apii dash giin. Bizaan igo omaa nanaamadabin megwaa omaa ayaawaad mawadishiwewaad maagizhaa gaye agwajiing gidaa-izhaa da-baa-odaminoyan.

[3] Asemaa omaa gidaa-asaa imaa nibiikaang dabwaa-bagizoyan ani-mikwenimad a'aw Manidoo eyaad imaa zaaga'iganiing maagizhaa gaye ziibiing. Gego anooj izhichigeken imaa baa-ayaayan i'iw zaaga'igan. Gidaa-manaaji'aa a'aw Manidoo imaa eyaad zaaga'iganiing. Ishke mewinzha gaawiin a'aw Anishinaabe gii-tapinesiin, gaawiin gaye gibwanaabaawesiin imaa nibiikaang onji apane weweni gii-asemaakawaawaad iniw Manidoon imaa zaaga'iganiing eyaanijin.

[4] Gego babaamendangen ingiw bineshiinyag owadiswaniwaan. Gego banaajitooken ingiw bineshiinyag iniw owaawanoomiwaan. Miinawaa gego inigaa'aaken ingiw banajaansag. Mikwendan ingoding gaye giin giniijaanisag giga-ayaawaag. Giga-bi-azheshkaagon ani-maazhichigeyan inigaatooyan i'iw bemaadiziimagak.

15 THIS IS THE WAY A CHILD SHOULD BE TAUGHT

[1] Do not be mean to your dog. The dog also has a spirit. Everything has a spirit that is here on earth.

[2] Do not interrupt adults when they are visiting. Sit here quietly while they are here visiting, maybe you can go outside and play.

[3] You should put tobacco in the water before you go swimming, remembering that spirit that exists in the lake or river. Do not raise heck or do foolish things while you are in the water. Treat that spirit in that lake respectfully. Years ago Anishinaabe people did not die or drown in the water, because they always put their tobacco in the lake or river.

[4] Do not bother the bird's nest. Do not destroy the bird's eggs. Do not hurt the little birdies. Remember that someday you will have your own children. What goes around comes around. If you destroy that which is alive, it will come back on you.

[5] Gego gizhibaabitawaaken a'aw gimishoomisinaan a'aw Manidoo dewe'igan megwaa baakishing. Ishke giishpin imaa bangishinan, gidaa-wenda-wiisagishin. Bizaan imaa nanaamadabin megwaa imaa ayaayan ani-aabajichigaazod a'aw gimishoomisinaan ani-niimi'idiiked a'aw Anishinaabe. Mikwendan mii imaa ishpiming ayaawaad ingiw Manidoog megwaa aabajichigaazod a'aw Manidoo-dewe'igan. Mii imaa wenzaabamaawaad wenjitawaawaad odanishinaabemiwaan megwaa niimi'idiikenid. Odaa-minwendaanaawaa ingiw Manidoog waabamikwaa bizaan imaa nanaamadabiyan weweni imaa bizindaman miinawaa weweni ganawaabiyan imaa enakamigak endazhi-niimi'idid a'aw Anishinaabe.

[6] Weweni bizindaw a'aw gechi-aya'aawid ani-waawiindamook gegoo. Gego ganage nakwetawaaken wenjida ani-naniibikimik ani-wanichigeyan gegoo, misawaa-go gikendaman egooyan. Gego ganage gegoo ikidoken.

[7] Gego baapinenimaaken ingiw Binesiwag miinawaa nichiiwak. Weweni a'aw gidasemaa gidaa-asaa da-nanaandomadwaa ingiw Binesiwag weweni da-ni-bimi-ayaawaad aaniindi-go a'aw Anishinaabe endanakiid. Gego dazhimaaken ingiw Binesiwag. Gego ikidoken, "Mii iw gii-pimi-ayaawaad ingiw Binesiwag, mii iw gii-ishkwaa-niiskaadak." Gaawiin anooj odaa-inaasiin iniw Binesiwan. Odaa-manaazomaan iniw Binesiwan. Ishke giishpin awiya i'iw ikidod, mii-go da-bi-azhegiiwewaapan miinawaa.

[8] Gego apane mamiikwaanidizoken. Mikwendan mii eta-go ingiw Manidoog wenjida gakina gegoo gekendangig, gaawiin giinawind. Gegapii-go gidaa-zhiingitaagoog ingiw Manidoog apane mamiikwaanidizoyan.

[5] Do not run around the ceremonial drums when they are open. If you fall while you are running, you can really hurt yourself. Sit quietly while you are at the ceremonial dances. Remember that those spirits are right above you when those drums are open. It is from there that they watch and listen to their people. The spirits will be happy to see you sitting quietly, listening carefully, and observing closely what is happening at the ceremonial dance.

[6] Listen to your elders when they give you advice or tell you something. Do not even think of talking back to your elders when they reprimand you for your behavior, even if you already know what you are being told. Do not even think of saying anything.

[7] Do not be disrespectful to the Thunder-beings and the storms. You could put your tobacco asking the Thunder-beings to go over in a good way wherever Anishinaabe live. Do not talk about the Thunder-beings. Do not say, "The Thunder-beings have gone by" or "The storm is over." Do not talk about the Thunder-beings. You have to be respectful when you speak to the Thunder-beings. If someone says that, they could come back again.

[8] Do not always brag about yourself. Remember that it is the spirits that are all knowledgeable, not us as human beings. The spirits could get tired of you always bragging about yourself.

[9] Zhawenim ingiw gechi-aya'aawijig. Gego baapi'aaken giishpin bishkwaabikinigewaad maagizhaa gaye zhiginidizowaad. Mikwendan ingoding gaye giin gidaa-gichi-aya'aaw.

[10] Gego nichiiwenimoken apane da-baa-inigaa'ad waaji'ad. Gaawiin ginwenzh bimaadizisiin nechiiwenimod.

[11] Zhawenim ingiw bakaan enaadizijig, miinawaa memaanjigozijig, naa gaye ayaabitawaadizijig. Mikwendan igo ogii-inenimigowaan iniw Manidoon i'iw akeyaa da-izhi-bimaadiziwaad, gegoo-go omaa da-onjikaamagad ge-gikinoo'amaagooyang.

[12] Giishpin maazhi-doodawad giwiiji-bimaadiziim, mii iniw mayaazhi-doodawimajin iniw Manidoon genawenimigowaajin. Ishke gaa-izhi-gikinoo'amaagoowiziyang gaawiin imaa daa-ayaasiin omaa akiing giishpin ayaawaasig iniw Manidoon zhewenimigojin miinawaa genawenimigojin.

[13] Gego agwajiing baa-odaminoken niibaa-dibik. Giishpin i'iw izhichigeyan gaawiin gikendaagwasinoon awenen imaa ge-baa-wiiji'ad.

[14] Gego zazaagiziken. Giishpin gegoo ayaaman gemaa gaye ziinzibaakwadoons aanind gidaa-miinaag giwiiji'aaganag. Ishke mikwendan ani-maamiigiweyan aanind i'iw eyaaman da-bi-azhegiiwemagad ingoding da-ni-manezisiwan gegoo.

[15] Gego gwiishkoshiken niibaa-dibik. Ingoji imaa awiya gidaa-nakwetaag da-zegi'ik.

[9] Have compassion for those that are elderly. Do not laugh at them if they should accidently pass gas or pee on themselves. Remember that someday you will also be old too.

[10] Do not be a bully hurting those who you play with. Bullies do not live long.

[11] Have compassion for those who were born differently, those who are physically disabled, and those who have an intellectual disability. Remember those spirits intended them to live that way; they were put on this earth to teach us something.

[12] If you harm your fellow Anishinaabe, it is actually those spirits that watch over them that you are doing harm too. What we have been taught is that a person would not be on this earth if we didn't have a spirit taking care of us and watching over us.

[13] Do not play outside during the night. If you would do that, it is hard telling who you would be playing with at night.

[14] Do not be stingy. If you have something such as candy, share it with your friends. Remember as you give things away, someday it will come back to you so that you are not without.

[15] Do not whistle at night. Somebody might answer your whistle and scare you.

[16] Apiitendan miinawaa manaajitoon i'iw wiisiniwin eshamigooyan wenjida gaa-miinigooyang anishinaabewiyang da-inanjigeyang. Weweni gidaa-doodaamin, gaawiin gidaa-nishwanaajitoosiimin, ishke ingiw Manidoog gigii-miinigonaanig i'iw akeyaa da-inanjigeyang.

[17] Gego baapi'aaken a'aw nebowa waasinid miinawaa wenda-nitaa-wiisinid naa go gaye a'aw wenda-nibaadizid. Gego anooj inaaken, gidaa-wenda-gagwaanisagendam gashkitoosig da-wiisinid awiya.

[18] Zhawenim a'aw eni-maazhi-doodook naa go gaye enigaa'ik, misawaa-go eni-doodook giwiiji-bimaadiziim booch igo da-zhawenimad. Ishke mii i'iw gaa-izhi-gikinoo'amaagoowiziyang anishinaabewiyang, misawaa-go eni-nisaad iniw besho enawemimang, mii-go booch da-zhawenimang imaa gaa-maazhichiged.

[19] Ani-naniibikimigooyan, gaawiin gimaazhi-doodaagoosiin. Gimino-doodaagoo, mii iw ge-ni-naadamaagooyan giniigaaniiming. Mii iw wenji-naniibikimind ani-abinoojiinyiwid awiya.

[20] Weweni bizindan i'iw akeyaa ezhi-gikinoo'amaagooyan, nebowa imaa ayaamagad ani-gikinoo'amaagooyan da-ni-manaajitooyan gegoo biinish gaye da-ni-manaaji'ad giwiiji-bimaadiziim. Ishke giishpin bizindanziwan ani-zhazhiibitaman i'iw akeyaa ezhi-gikinoo'amaagooyan, ishke mii i'iw ge-ni-izhiwebiziyan giniigaaniiming. Gaawiin gegoo gidaa-ni-manaajitoosiin miinawaa wawaaj igo gaawiin gidaa-ni-apiitenimaasiin giwiiji-bimaadiziim, mii-go gegapii-go da-ni-maazhi-doodawad a'aw giwiiji-bimaadiziim. Gaawiin anishaa imaa gigii-miinigoowizisiimin i'iw akeyaa ezhi-gikinoo'amawind ani-nitaawigi'ind a'aw Anishinaabe-abinoojiinh, mii iw ge-ni-naadamaagod oniigaaniiming.

[16] Value the food you are being fed and treat it respectfully, especially those foods we have been given to eat. Treat it respectfully and do not waste it, since it was the spirits that gave us those foods to eat.

[17] Do not laugh at those who eat a lot, those who love to eat, and those who have big appetites. Do not criticize them; you would feel terrible if these people were not able to eat.

[18] Forgive those who do you wrong and those who hurt you, regardless of whatever a person may do to you; you still have to have compassion for them. That's what we were taught as Anishinaabe; even if a person was to kill our close relative, we still have to have compassion for them.

[19] When you are being disciplined, they are not doing wrong to you. They are being good to you and giving you what will help you in your future. That is why a child is scolded.

[20] Listen carefully to what you are being taught; you are being taught to treat all things with respect and all people with respect. If you do not listen and let what you are being taught go in one ear and out the other, this is how you will live your life from here on out. If you do not respect anything or have respect for your fellow man, sooner or later you will hurt somebody. There was a reason we were given these teachings to be utilized with our children. It is what will help them in their future.

[21] Giishpin awiya manezid maagizhaa gaye ani-gagwaadagitood, gidaa-zhawenimaa da-ni-naadamawad. Ishke ani-mino-doodawang ani-naadamawang a'aw giwiiji-bimaadiziiminaan, ingoding daa-bi-azhegiiwemagad aazhita da-ni-naadamaagoowiziyang gaye giinawind.

[22] Gego nishwanaajitooken giwiiyaw da-ni-aabajitooyan i'iw minikwewin miinawaa anooj ani-aabajitood a'aw bemaadizid enigaa'igod. Gaawiin omaa gigii-asigoosiin omaa akiing da-ni-nishwanaajitooyan giwiiyaw i'iw akeyaa. Gakina bebezhig a'aw bemaadizid iniw Manidoon ayaamagadini gaa-onji-asigod omaa akiing. Gegoo-go ogii-inenimigoon iniw Manidoon da-ni-izhichiged megwaa omaa bibizhaagiid omaa akiing. Mii iw ge-nandawaabandaman ani-mikaman, mii i'iw ge-ni-biminizha'aman megwaa omaa bibizhaagiiyan omaa akiing.

[23] Ayaangwaamizin da-gikinoo'amaagoziyan miinawaa weweni da-bizindaman ezhi-gikinoo'amaagooyan. Ishke ani-wawiingeziyan omaa gikinoo'amaagoziyan, mii i'iw ge-ni-aabajitooyan giniigaaniiming da-ni-bami'idizoyan naa gaye giniijaanisag.

[24] Weweni bizindan ani-gikinoo'amaagooyan i'iw akeyaa gaa-izhi-wiindamawind a'aw Anishinaabe da-ni-bimiwidood i'iw bimaadiziwin. Mii i'iw da-ni-naadamaagooyan giniigaaniiming da-ni-baazhidaakonigooyan. Ingoding giniigaaniiming gidaa-ni-aabajitoon i'iw akeyaa gaa-izhi-gikinoo'amaagooyan, ishke aazhita gidaa-ni-gikinoo'amawaag giniijaanisag. Ishke ani-bizindanziwan weweni, ingoding giniigaaniiming mii iw ge-ikidoyan, "Apegish weweni gii-pizindamaambaan owapii aana-gii-gikinoo'amaagooyaan a'aw Anishinaabe gaa-miinigoowizid i'iw akeyaa da-ni-izhi-bimaadizid."

[21] If someone is without or is having a difficult time, you should have compassion for them and help them out. If we are good to our fellow man and reach out to help them, someday it will come back to us when we are in need ourselves.

[22] Do not waste your life by using alcohol or drugs. You were not put on this earth to waste your life away by using alcohol and drugs. Each one of us has been put on this earth for a reason. There is something those spirits want us to accomplish while we are here. You need to find out your purpose in life and pursue it while you are here on earth.

[23] Work hard at pursuing your education and listen carefully to what you are being taught. If you do well at school, you will be able to use it in your future to support yourself and your family.

[24] Listen carefully to the teachings. Anishinaabe have been taught to live a good life. That is what will help you in your future and carry you over those hurdles in life. Sometime in your future, you can put those teachings to use and pass them on to your children. If you do not listen, someday in your future you will be saying, "I wish I would have listened more carefully on those teachings of how to live a good life as Anishinaabe."

[25] Gego mamooken a'aw Chi-mookomaan i'iw akeyaa ezhitwaad.
Gego gidaa-wii-wayezhimigosiin a'aw wayaabishkiiwed.
Gigii-miinigonaanig ingiw Manidoog anishinaabewiyang
ge-izhitwaayang. Geget ingiw Manidoog ogii-shawenimaawaan
inow odanishinaabemiwaan. Geget onaajiwan gaa-izhi-
miinigoowiziyang da-ni-bimiwidooyang bimaadiziyang.
Giishpin a'aw Anishinaabe ani-maamood a'aw Chi-mookomaan
ezhitwaad, ishke gegoo izhiwebizid, gaawiin da-izhaasiin iwidi
gidinawemaaganinaanig eni-izhaawaad ani-aanjikiiwaad.

[26] Gego nisidizoken. Ishke ingiw Manidoog gii-inaakonigewag
i'iwapii ge-ni-aanjikiiyan. Gaawiin giin gidaa-inaakonigesiin
owapii. Ishke giishpin nisidizoyan, gaawiin gidaa-izhaasiin
iwidi ezhaawaad ingiw gidinawemaaganinaanig ani-
aanjikiiwaad. Mii imaa da-ni-baataashinan opimekana
da-ni-maamiijiyan iniw ojiibikoon. Gaawiin dash gidaa-ni-
de-dagoshimoonosiin eni-izhaawaad gidinawemaaganinaanig
gaagwiinawaabaminaagoziwaad omaa akiing.

[27] Weweni bizindan aadizookaagooyan. Gego nibaaken
megwaa aadizookaagooyan. Ishke gegoo-go omaa gidaa-
ina'oonwewiz ani-bizindaman inow aadizookaanan,
ishke ingiw Manidoog imaa eni-dazhinjigaazojig.
Gidaa-zhawenimigoog.

[28] Gego imaa mikwamiing odaminoken niibaa-dibik. Gidaa-
nagishkawaa a'aw Bebookawe megwaa imaa baa-odaminoyan
mikwamiing niibaa-dibik.

[29] Gego gimoodiken. Gaawiin gidaa-niigaaniisiin gimoodiyan.
Eshkam igo nawaj awashime gidaa-ni-wanitoon gegoo nawaj igo
da-apiitendaagwak apii dash i'iw gaa-kimoodiyan ge-wanitooyan.

[25] Do not take the white man's way of life or his religion. Do not let him deceive you into adopting his belief system. The spirits gave us as Anishinaabe our own belief system and way of life. The spirits had a lot of compassion for the Anishinaabe. They gave us a beautiful way of life and a belief system on how to live our lives. If an Anishinaabe takes the white man's religion, when he dies he will not go to where our relatives go when they leave this world.

[26] Do not commit suicide. The spirits have decided when we will change worlds. It is not up to you to decide when you will change worlds. If you commit suicide, you will not go to where our relatives go when they change worlds. You will get stuck alongside that path eating roots. You will not reach that destination where our relatives go when they change worlds.

[27] Listen carefully when you are being told Winter Legends. Do not fall asleep while you are being told these stories. You could be gifted in one way or another if you listen carefully; the characters that are being talked about are spirits. They may gift you with something.

[28] Do not play on the ice at night. You could meet up with the *Bebookawe* while playing out there at night.

[29] Do not steal. You will not get ahead by stealing. You will eventually lose more than what you have gained from stealing.

[30] Gego gaagaawenimaaken a'aw giwiiji-anishinaabem. Gidaa-miigwechiwendam miinawaa gidaa-minawaanigwendam ani-noondaman a'aw giwiiji-anishinaabem ani-mamiikwaanind miinawaa ani-debibidood gegoo o'ow akeyaa ge-ni-izhi-niigaaniid.

[31] Gego maazhi-doodawaaken ingiw asiniig. Ishke ingiw asiniig Manidoog ingiw. Gimishoomisinaanig izhi-wiinaawag. Gego imaa nibiikaang apaginaaken ingiw asiniig. Gego apaginaaken asiniig ogijayi'ii imaa nibiing da-onji-gwaashkwaniwaad.

[32] Gego gitimiken naa gaye gego bagandiziken. Gidaa-nandawaabandaan anooj gegoo ge-dazhiikaman. Gidaa-naadamaage anooj gegoo imaa da-naadamawadwaa gigitiziimag. Ishke a'aw Anishinaabe ishkweyaang gaa-ayaad geget gii-kinzhizhawizi. Gaawiin bizaan gii-nanaamadabisiin. Geget ogii-wenda-gichi-apiitenimaawaan miinawaa ogii-mamiikwaanaawaan inow Anishinaaben gaa-kinzhizhawizinijin.

[33] Geget a'aw Anishinaabe mewinzha gii-kinzhizhawizi. Mii imaa gii-gikinawaadendaagwak gaa-inaajimotawid a'aw mindimooyenyiban gaa-nitaawigi'id. Mii imaa gii-tazhindang gaa-onji-biindaakwed, mii imaa gii-wiindamawid gii-sagaswaad iko, "Ishke dash gaawiin nigii-minwendanziin wanishkwe'igoyaan megwaa imaa anokiiyaan, akawe imaa gii-ni-nanaamadabiyaan gii-sagaswaayaan gii-wanishkwe'igoyaan megwaa imaa anokiiyaan. Mii dash gaa-izhi-moonendamaan, giishpin biindaakweyaan gaawiin inga-wanishkwe'igosiin megwaa imaa anokiiyaan. Mii dash imaa gaa-onji-mamooyaan biindaakweyaan dash noongom."

[30] Do not be jealous or envious of your fellow Anishinaabe. You should be grateful and happy when you hear your fellow Anishinaabe being praised or receiving something that helps them get ahead in life.

[31] Do not harm the rocks. These rocks have a spirit within them. They are known as our grandfathers. Do not throw these rocks in the water. Do not skip the rocks across the top of the water.

[32] Do not be lazy and worthless. You can look for something to work on. You can help your parents out with different things. Our Anishinaabe in the past were hard workers. They did not sit still. They really admired the Anishinaabe who were hard workers.

[33] Anishinaabe were definitely hard working, long ago. This was obvious in what that old lady told me. She talked about why she chews now. She told me that she smoked at one time, "I did not like to be interrupted in my work, I didn't like the idea that I had to stop and sit down to have a smoke. I realized that if I took up snuff chewing it would not interrupt my work. That is why I chew snuff today."

[34] Mii iw gaa-inaajimotawid a'aw mindimooyenyiban gaa-nitaawigi'id. Mii gaye ayaapii gaa-ikidod, "Mii imaa wenjida ojaanimiziyaan wanishkwe'id ninjiid." Mii iw gaa-tazhindang mii wenjida owapii bagamishkaagozid waakaa'igaansing wii-o-zaaga'ang. Gaawiin ogii-minwendanziin akawe imaa ani-noogitaad waakaa'igaansing izhaad megwaa ojaanimizid imaa anokiid. Ogii-wanishkwe'igon. Mii imaa gii-wiindamaaged gaa-izhi-minwendang anokiid miinawaa gaa-izhi-ginzhizhawizid.

[35] Gagwe-gikendan da-nitaa-jiibaakweyan. Ishke gikendaman da-nitaa-jiibaakweyan, gaawiin memwech gidaa-apenimosiin awiya da-jiibaakook giniigaaniiming.

[36] Giishpin ani-gagwaadagitooyan da-ni-boodaweyan maagizhaa-go gaye nitaa-boodawesiwan, da-gitimishki a'aw ikwe ge-ni-wiij'ayaawad.

[37] Giishpin nanaapaadakizineyan, giga-ni-nagishkawaa gidoodem ani-bimi-ayaayan i'iw miikana.

[38] Giishpin napaazi-zagaakwa'aman gibabagiwayaan, mii iko gaa-inind awiya, ginoodendam.

[39] Gego waasa imaa baa-ayaaken azhigwa biboong. Besho-go imaa gidaa-wii-ayaa jiigayi'ii imaa endaayan. Ishke gezika daa-wenda-niiskaadad, gaawiin gidaa-waabisiin waasa ezhi-niiskaadak. Mii dash imaa da-baa-wanishinamban. Gaawiin gidaa-mikanziin weweni da-giiweyamban.

[34] That is what that old lady who raised me told me. She would also say, "It seems that when I am really busy, that is when my butt would interrupt me." It was when she was really busy that she felt the need to go to the outhouse. She didn't like to be interrupted by the need to go to the outhouse, especially when she was busy doing something. By telling this, she emphasized how she enjoyed being a hard worker.

[35] Work at learning how to cook. If you learn how to cook, you will not have to rely on someone to cook for you in your future.

[36] If you have difficulties making a fire or just do not know how to make a fire, you will have a lazy wife.

[37] If you put your shoes on the wrong feet, you will run into the animal from your clan on the road.

[38] If you button your shirt wrong, they used to say, you must have someone on your mind that you are attracted to.

[39] Do not go far in the wintertime. Stay close to your home. A storm or the wind can come up quickly. You would not be able to see far, and that is where you could get lost and not be able to find your way home.

[40] Gego daanginangen naa-go gaye gego dazhiikangen
i'iw debendanziwan wenjida ingoji baa-ayaayan baa-
mawadishiweyan. Mii iko gaa-igooyaan gii-naniibikimigooyaan
gii-ni-bizindanziwaan o'ow akeyaa gaa-izhi-gikinoo'amaagooyaan
da-ni-dazhiikanziwaan i'iw debendanziwaan, "Ishke giishpin
awiya ojiid waabandaman etenig, mii-go mamooyamban da-ni-
daanginaman da-ni-zinigobidooyan mii-go ge-izhichigeyamban.

[41] Gego dazhiikangen gego gaye daanginangen iniw Manidoo-
aabajichiganan debendangin awiya.

[42] Gego ani-gagwedweken megwaa imaa ani-manidoowichiged
a'aw Anishinaabe. Gomaapii gidaa-ni-gikendaan eni-izhichiged
a'aw Anishinaabe omaa ani-asemaaked. Mii iko a'aw Chi-
mookomaan ezhichiged. Gego giin izhichigeken.

[43] Gego aabidaanagidoongen naa gego onzaamidoongen.
Mii iw Chi-mookomaan ezhichiged. Dibishkoo gaawiin a'aw
wayaabishkiiwed ominwendanziin banganinig. Mii dash imaa
anooj ani-gaagwiinawi-ikidod ani-nishwanaaji-ikidod.

[40] Do not touch or handle those things that do not belong to you, especially when you are out visiting. They used to give me heck and scold me when I would not listen to this teaching, touching something that did not belong to me, "If you saw someone's genitals sitting there, you would probably touch them or rub them, that's probably what you would do."

[41] Do not bother or touch the sacred items that belong to someone else.

[42] Do not ask questions during the course of a ceremony. In time you will know what an Anishinaabe is doing as he puts tobacco. That is something that a white man would do. Do not do that.

[43] Do not talk too much or be mouthy. That is what a white man does. It is as if he is uncomfortable with silence. It is then that he tries to find something to say and says meaningless things.

GLOSSARY

The glossary presented here mainly follows the conventions set forth by the Ojibwe People's Dictionary (online). The abbreviations employed for the various parts of speech are given here:

adv conj	conjunctive adverb
adv deg	degree adverb
adv dub	dubitative adverb
adv gram	grammatical adverb
adv inter	interrogative adverb
adv loc	locational adverb
adv man	manner adverb
adv neg	negative adverb
adv num	number adverb
adv pred	predicative adverb
adv qnt	quantitative adverb
adv tmp	temporal adverb
na	animate noun
na-v	animate participle
nad	dependent animate noun
nad-pret	dependent animate noun preterit mode
name pers	personal name
name place	place name
ni	inanimate noun
ni-v	inanimate participle
nid	dependent inanimate noun
pc asp	aspectual particle
pc disc	discourse particle
pc emph	emphatic particle
pron dem	demonstrative pronoun
pron dub	dubitative pronoun

pron indf	indefinite pronoun
pron inter	interrogative pronoun
pron per	personal pronoun
pron psl	pausal pronoun
pv dir	direction preverb, pv2
pv lex	lexical preverb, pv4
pv rel	relative preverb, pv3
pv tns	tense/mode preverb, pv1
qnt num	uninflected number
vai+o	animate intransitive verb with object
vai	animate intransitive verb
vai2	animate transitive verb (class 2, -m endings)
vii	inanimate intransitive verb
vta	animate transitive verb
vti	inanimate transitive verb
vti2	inanimate transitive verb (class 2, -oon endings)
vti3	inanimate transitive verb (class 3, -in endings)
vti4	inanimate transitive verb (class 4, -aan endings)

Other abbreviations

h/	animate object or possessor; him, her, it (animate); his, hers
s/he	animate subject: she, he, it (animate)
h/self	himself or herself
pl	plural

abinoojiinh *na* child

abinoojiinyens *na* infant

abinoojiinyensiwi *vai* s/he is a baby

abinoojiinyiwi *vai* s/he is a child

abiichigaazo *vai* a wake is held for h/ (by someone), "they" hold a wake for h/

achigaade *vii* it is put in a certain place (by someone), "they" put it in a certain place

achigaazo *vai* s/he is put in a certain place (by someone); "they" put h/ in a certain place

agana *adv qnt* not to the extent; less

agaaming *adv loc* on the other side of a body of water (a lake, a river), across a body of water (a lake, a river)

agoojigaade *vii* it is hung (by someone), "they" hang it

agwajiing *adv loc* outside, outdoors

agwaawebin *vta* throw h/ out of water

a'aw *pron dem* that; *animate singular demonstrative; also* **aw**

Ajidiwaashiikwe *name pers* Nancy Churchill

akakanzhe *ni* charcoal, coals

akawe *adv tmp* first (in time sequence), first of all, for now

akeyaa *adv tmp* in the direction of, that way

aki *ni* earth, land, ground, country

akiwenzii *na* old man

ako- *pv rel* since; as long as

akwaandawaazh *vta* climb on h/; rape h/

Amikogaabawiikwe *name pers* Julie Shingobe

amo /amw-/ *vta* eat h/

anamikaw *vta* greet h/, welcome h/

anang *na* star

anaakan *ni* a mat

ani- *pv dir* going away, going along, in progress, on the way, coming up in time; *also* **ni-**

animosh *na* dog

anishaa *adv man* just for nothing; without purpose; just for fun; not really

Anishinaabe *na* Ojibwe, person, human, Indian (in contrast to non-Indians)

Anishinaabe-abinoojiinh *na* an Ojibwe child

anishinaabe-zhiiwaagamizigan *ni* maple syrup

Anishinaabekwe *na* an Indian woman; an Ojibwe woman

anishinaabemo *vai* s/he speaks Ojibwe

anishinaabemotaadiwag *vai* they speak Ojibwe to each other

anishinaabewi *vai* s/he is Ojibwe, is human, Indian (in contrast to non-Indians)

anishinaabewinikaade *vii* it is called in Ojibwe

anishinaabewinikaazo *vai* s/he is called in Ojibwe

anishinaabewinikaazowin *ni* an Ojibwe name

aniibiish *ni* tea

anokii *vii* s/he works

anooj *adv qnt* various, all kinds

anoozh /anooN-/ *vta* ask h/ to do something, hire h/, give an order to h/, commission h/

apagizom *vta* send h/ (by voice) (e.g., tobacco)

apagizondamaw *vta* send (it) to h/ (by voice) (e.g., tobacco)

apagizonjigaade *vii* it is sent (by voice); "they" send it (by voice) (e.g., food, *inanimate* items)

apagizh /apagiN-/ *vta* throw h/

apa'iwe *vai* s/he runs away from people to a certain place

apane *adv tmp* always, all the time, continually

apegish *adv pred* I wish that . . .

apenimo *vta* s/he relies on something, depends on something

apigaabawi *vai+o* s/he relies on (it) for spiritual support

apinikaazo *vai* s/he is named after somebody (e.g., a spirit, a manidoo)

apii *adv tmp* when, then, at the time

apiitendamaw *vta* value h/ to a certain extent, appreciate h/, respect h/

apiitendan *vti* value it to a certain extent, appreciate it

apiitendaagozi *vai* s/he is valued so high, ranks so high, is so important, is worthy, is appreciated

apiitendaagwad *vii* it is valued so high, ranks so high, is so important, is worthy, is appreciated

apiitenim *vta* be proud of h/ to a certain extent, feel about h/ to a certain extent

asabikeshiinh-wanii'igan *ni* dream catcher

asemaa *na* tobacco

asemaa-onaagan *ni* tobacco dish

asemaakaw *vta* make an offering of tobacco to h/

asemaake *vai* s/he makes a tobacco offering

asin *na* a rock

asham *vta* feed (it) to h/

ashamoonsi *vai+o* s/he feeds people

ashange *vai* s/he feeds people, serves food

ashi /aS-/ *vta* put h/ in a certain place

ashi-bezhig *adv num* eleven

ashi-naanan *adv num* fifteen

atamaw *vta* put something in a certain place for h/

ataagewigamig *ni* casino

ate *vii* it is in a certain place

atemagad *vii* it is in a certain place

atoon *vti2* put it in a certain place

awasayi'ii *adv loc* beyond it; on the other side of it

awashime *adv qnt* much more

awedi bezhig *pron dem* that other one over there

awegonen *pron inter* what. *inanimate interrogative*

awegonen danaa *adv inter* what the heck?

awegwen igo *pron dub* whoever

awenen *pron inter* who. *animate interrogative*

awesiinh *na* wild animal

awiya *pron indf* somebody, anybody. *animate indefinite*

aya'aa *pron psl* I don't remember who, I don't know who

aya'aansiwi *vai* s/he is young

ayaa *vai* s/he is (in a certain place); *with a lexical preverb* s/he is in a certain state; *with a directional preverb* s/he moves in a certain way

ayaamagad *vii* it is (in a certain place); *with a lexical preverb* it is in a certain state; *with a directional preverb* it moves in a certain way

ayaan /ayaam-/ *vti4* have it, own it

ayaangwaamim *vta* encourage h/, warn h/, caution h/

ayaangwaamitoon *vti2* carefully do it, cautiously do it

ayaangwaamizi *vai* s/he is careful, cautious

ayaapii *adv tmp* every once in a while, every so often

ayaaw *vta* have h/, own h/

azhegiiwe *vai* s/he goes or comes back, returns

azhegiiwemagad *vii* it goes or comes back, it returns

azhegiiwewizh *vta* return h/

azhenizha'w *vta* send h/ back

azheshkaw *vta* [inverse] it comes back to you; (e.g., giga-bi-azheshkaagon, It [karma] will come back to you)

azheyaajim *vta* retell a story of h/

azhigwa *adv tmp* now, at this time, already, then

aabajichigaade *vii* it is used (by someone), "they" use it

aabajichigaazo *vai* s/he is used (by someone), "they" use h/

aabaji' *vta* use h/

aabajitoon *vti2* use it

aabidaanagidoon *vai* s/he talks continually

aabiding *adv tmp* once, at one time

aabiji- *pv lex* continually, constantly

aabita-biboon *vii* it is midwinter

aabitawaadizi *vai* s/he has an intellectual disability

aadizookaw *vta* tell a sacred story (winter legend) to h/

aadizookaan *na* a winter legend; sacred story

aadizooke *vai* s/he tells a sacred story (winter legend)

aakozi *vai* s/he is sick, is ill

aakoziwin *ni* a sickness, an illness, a disease

aana- *pv lex* in vain, without result

aanawendan *vti* dislike it, reject it, discount it, find it unsatisfactory or inferior

aanawenim *vta* dislike h/, reject h/, find h/ unsatisfactory or inferior

aanawenindizo *vai* s/he finds h/self unsatisfactory or inferior

aanind *adv qnt* some

aaningodinong *adv temp* sometimes, occasionally

aaniin *adv inter* how?, why?, in what way?

aaniin igo apii *adv tmp* whenever

aaniindi *adv inter* where?

aaniindi-go *adv loc* wherever

aaniish naa *adv man* after all, well now; you see

aanjikii *vai* s/he changes worlds

aano-go *adv man* anyhow, although, despite, but; *also* **aanawi**

aanoodizi *vai* s/he desires, s/he is determined

aapiji *adv deg* very, quite

aasamisag *ni* a wall

aawi *vai* s/he is a certain thing or being

aayaabajitoon *vti2* use it. Reduplication of **aabajitoon**

aayaajim *vta* tell a story of h/. Reduplication of **aajim**

aazhikwe *vai* s/he screams

aazhita *adv man* in return

Aazhoomog *name place* Mille Lacs Reservation village on St. Croix River Minnesota border

ba- *pv* this way, here, hither (bi- *under IC*)

babagiwayaan *ni* shirt

babaa- *pv dir* going about

babaa-ayaa *vai* s/he is around, wanders about

babaamaadizi *vai* s/he travels about

babaamendan *vti* be bothered by it

babaamibatoo *vai* s/he runs about

babaamitaw *vta* pay attention to what h/ says, worry about what h/ says

babiiwaamagad *vii* it is tiny

babiiwizhiinyiwi *vai* s/he is tiny

badakidemagad *vii* it sticks up, stands up (from a surface)

bagakendam *vai2* s/he has a clear mind, is aware

bagamagoode *vii* it arrives hanging

bagamishkaagozi *vai* s/he is overcome

bagandizi *vai* s/he is lazy, is incompetent

bagida'waa *vai* s/he fishes (with a net), sets net

bagidin *vta* set h/ down, offer h/, release h/, let h/ go, allow h/

bagijige *vai* s/he makes an offering

bagijwebinan *vti* release it quickly, throw it down quickly

bagizo *vai* s/he goes swimming

bagosenim *vta* wish for h/, hope for h/

bagwaj *adv loc* in the wilderness, out in the woods

Bagwaj-inini *name pers* The Big Man in the Woods (a Manidoo that lives in the woods and appears as a man)

bakaan *adv man* different

bakaanad *vii* it is different

bakaanige *vai* she is secluded at first menses

bakaanigondaagan *vai* he has a different voice (e.g., puberty change)

bakwajisemagad *vii* it comes out or off of something

bami'idizo *vai* s/he supports, provides for h/ self

banajaans *na* a baby bird, a nestling

banaajitoon *vti2* spoil it, damage it

bangan *vii* it is peaceful, is quiet

bangishimo *vai* the sun sets

bangishin *vai* s/he falls

bangiiwagizi *vai* there is a little bit of h/; *plural* there are few of them

bapagone'an *vti* make a hole in it (using something).
   Reduplication of **bagone'an**

bapagoshkaamagad *vii* it has holes

bashkwegino-makizinens *ni* buckskin moccasin

bawaajigan *ni* a dream, a vision

bawaajige *vai* s/he has dreams

bazigwii *vai* s/he stands up

baa-ayaa *vai* s/he is around, wanders about

baabii'o *vai* s/he keeps waiting

baabiitawayi'ii *adv loc* in-between

baakishim *vta* leave h/ uncovered

baakishin *vai* s/he is left open, left uncovered

baapi' *vta* laugh at h/

baapinendan *vti* be disrespectful to it

baapinenim *vta* make fun of h/, lack respect for h/

baataasin *vii* it is stuck

baataashin *vai* s/he gets stuck

baazhidaakokii *vai* s/he steps over

baazhidaakon *vta* carry h/ over

baazhidaakonigoowizi *vai* s/he will be carried over something
   (by a higher power)

bebakaan *adv man* all different

bebezhig *adv num* one by one

Bebookawe *name pers* a Manidoo who looks like a man engulfed
   in flames

besho *adv loc* near, close

bezhig *adv num* one

bezhigwan *vii* it is the same

bi- *pv dir* this way, here, hither

bi-izhaa *vai* s/he comes

bibizhaagii *vai* s/he lives in a certain place

biboon *vii* it is winter

biboonagad *vii* it is a winter, it (a year) passes

bijiinag *adv tmp* after awhile, recently, just now

bikwak *ni* an arrow
bikwaakwad *ni* a ball
bimaadizi *vai* s/he lives, is alive
bimaadiziwin *ni* life
bimaadiziimagad *vii* it is alive
bimi- *pv dir* along, going along, going by, going past, on the way
bimi-ayaa *vai* s/he goes, travels along
bimi-ayaamagad *vii* it goes along, by, past
biminizha'an *vti* chase it along, pursue it
bimisemagad *vii* it (time) goes along, passes
bimiwidoon *vti2* carry it along, take it along; carry it on, conduct it
bimiwizh /bimiwiN-/ *vta* carry h/ along, take h/ along
Binesiwag *na-pl* Thunder beings; Manidoog
bineshiinh *na* a bird
bishkwaabikinige *vai* s/he accidently passes gas, farts
bitaakoshkan *vti* bump into it
bizaan *adv man* quiet, quietly, still, at peace
bizaanishin *vai* s/he lies still
bizindam *vai2* s/he listens
bizindan *vti* listen to it
bizindaw *vta* listen to h/
biibiiyens *na* a baby
biindaakoodoon *vti2* offer tobacco to it
biindaakoojige *vai* s/he makes an offering of tobacco
biindaakoozh /biindaakooN-/ *vta* make an offering of tobacco to h/
biindaakwe *vai* s/he chews tobacco
biindig *adv loc* inside
biindigadoon *vti2* bring it inside, take it inside
biindigazh /biindigaN-/ *vta* bring h/ inside, take h/ inside
biindige *vai* s/he enters, goes inside, comes inside
biingeyendam *vai2* s/he is baffled, amazed, dumbfounded
biinish *adv gram* until, up to; continuing on
biinish gaye *adv man* and also

biinizikaa *adv man* suddenly; spontaneously; for no reason

biinji- *pv loc* inside

biinji-odaabaan *adv loc* inside the car

biinji-wiigiwaam *adv loc* inside the wigwam

biinjibajige *vai* s/he puts gas in a car

biinjina *adv loc* inside the body

biizikaagan *ni* item of clothing

biizikoon /biizikooN/ *vta* dress h/, put clothes on h/

booch *adv man* it is necessary, it is certain, you have to

boodawe *vai* s/he builds a fire

boonitoon *vti2* leave it alone, quit it

boozikanaagan *ni* bowl

Bwaan-akiing *ni* Dakota country

Bwaanikwe *na* a Dakota woman

chi- *pv lex* big, great; *also* **gichi-**

Chi-mookomaan *na* white man

Chi-mookomaani-mashkikiwinini *ni* a white doctor (in contrast to traditional healer)

da- *pv tns* future tense

da- *pv dir* that, so that, in order to; *future and modal prefix in unchanged conjunct; also* **ji-**

dabazhish *adv* low, down low

dabwaa- *pv tns* before

dadibaajim *vta* tell of h/. Reduplication of **dibaajim**

dagonigaade *vii* it is added, mixed in (by someone), "they" add, mix it in

dagoshimoonagad *vii* it arrives

dagoshimoono *vai* s/he arrives

dagoshimoono' *vta* get h/ to h/ destination

dagoshin *vai* s/he arrives

dakobizh /dakobiN-/ *vta* tie, bind h/

dakokaazh /dakokaaN-/ *vta* step on h/

dakon *vta* hold, take hold of h/

danakamigad *vii* it (an event) takes place, happens in a certain place

danakamigizi *vai* s/he has an event in a certain place

danakii *vai* s/he lives in a certain place

danizi *vai* s/he is in a certain place

dapaabam *vta* peek (through an opening) at h/, look through an opening at h/

dapine *vai* s/he suffers in a certain place, s/he dies in a certain place

daso-biboonagazi *vai* s/he is a certain number of years old; is so many years old

dash *adv conj* and; *also* **idash**

datazhinjigaazo *vai* s/he talked about, discussed (by someone), "they" talk about, discuss h/. Reduplication of **dazhinjigaazo**

dazhi- *pv rel* in a certain place, of a certain place, there

dazhim *vta* talk about h/, discuss h/

dazhindan *vti* talk about it, discuss it

dazhinjigaazo *vai* s/he talked about, discussed (by someone), "they" talk about, discuss h/

dazhitaa *vai* s/he spends time in a certain place

dazhiikan *vti* work at it, on it; be involved, occupied, engaged with it

dazhiikaw *vta* work at h/; be involved, occupied, engaged with h/

daa *vai* s/he lives in a certain place

daa- *pv* would, could, should, can, might *modal*

daanginan *vti* touch it (with hand)

daangizideshimoono' *vta* make h/ touch h/ feet to something

daangizideshkan *vti* touch it with h/ feet

de- *pv lex* sufficient, suitable, enough

debibidoon *vti2* grab, catch, get hold of it

debibizh /debibiN-/ *vta* grab, catch, get hold of h/

debinaak *adv man* carelessly, half-heartedly

debwetaw *vta* believe, agree with, obey h/

dedebinawe *adv man* by oneself, inherently, actual, biological

desapabiwin *ni* a bench

dewe'igan *na* a drum

dewe'igaans *na* a small drum, hand drum

dibaabam *vta* check up on h/

dibaajim *vta* tell of h/

dibaajimo *vai* s/he tells, tells a story

dibaajimowin *ni* a story; a narrative

dibendan *vti* control it, be the master of it, own it, earn it

dibendaagozi *vai* s/he belongs, is a member

dibiki-giizis *na* moon

dibishkoo *adv man* just like, even, equal, direct

dikinaagan *ni* a cradleboard

ditibishin *vai* s/he rolls

doodan *vti* do something to 1t

doodaw *vta* do something to h/

doodooshaaboo *ni* milk

eko- *pv rel* since, a certain length, as long as (ako- *under IC*)

emikwaanens *ni* spoon

endasing *adv tmp* every time

endaso-giizis *adv tmp* every month

endaso-giizhik *adv tmp* every day

endazhi- *pv rel* in a certain place, of a certain place, there (dazhi *under IC*)

endazhi-apagiji-ziigwebinigeng *ni-v* the garbage can, trash can

eni- *pv dir* coming up to in time; going away; in progress; on the way (ani- *under IC*)

eshkam *adv deg* gradually, more and more, less and less

eta *adv deg* only

ezhi- *pv rel* in a certain way; in a certain place; thus; so; there (izhi- *under IC*)

ga- *pv tns* future tense

gabe-biboon *adv tmp* all winter

gabe-bimaadizi *vai* s/he lives a full life (past one hundred years old)

gagaanwaanikwe *vai* s/he has long hair

gagaanzom *vta* persuade, urge, convince h/

gagiibaadizi *vai* s/he is foolish, is silly

gagwaadaginikaazo *vai* s/he has a difficult name

gagwaadagitoo *vai* s/he has a hard time, suffers

gagwaanisagendam *vai2* s/he thinks terrible, horrible, disgusting; s/he is horrified

gagwe- *pv lex* try

gagwedwe *vai* s/he asks questions, s/he inquires

gagwejim *vta* ask h/

gakina *adv qnt* all

ganabaj *adv man* one thinks that, maybe

ganawaabam *vta* look at, watch h/

ganawaabandan *vti* look at it, watch it

ganawaabi *vai* s/he looks, watches

ganawendamaage *vai* s/he takes care of things for people

ganawendan *vti* take care of, protect, keep it

ganawenim *vta* take care of h/, watch over h/

ganawenindizo *vai* s/he takes care of h/ self, is self-reliant

ganawenjigaade *vii* it is taken care of, protected, kept (by someone), "they" take care of, protect, keep it

ganawenjigaazo *vai* s/he is taken care of, protected, kept (by someone), "they" take care of, protect, keep h/

ganoodamaw *vta* speak for h/

ganoodamaadizo *vai* s/he speaks for h/ self

ganoodamaage *vai* s/he speaks for people

gashkapijigaazo *vai* s/he is wrapped and tied in a bundle (by someone); "they" wrap and tie h/ in a bundle

gashkapizh /gashkapiN-/ *vta* tie / shut, tie h/ up in a bundle

gashkibijigaazo *vai* s/he is wrapped and tied in a bundle (by someone), "they" tie and wrap h/ in a bundle

gashkigwaadan *vti* sew it

gashkigwaaso *vai* s/he sews

gashki'ewizi *vai* s/he is able to do something, is capable

gashkitoon *vti2* be able to do it, succeed at it, manage it

gayat *adv tmp* formerly, previously, some time ago

gaye *adv conj* as for, also, too, and

gaa- *pv tns* [past tense prefix under initial change]

Gaa-biboonike *name pers* Manidoo in the snow; snow

gaabige *adv tmp* already; so soon; so suddenly; in such a short time

gaagaawenim *vta* be jealous of h/. Reduplication of **gaawenim**

Gaagebiikwe *name pers* Misko Binayshi

Gaagige-minawaanigoziwining *name place* Land of Everlasting Happiness

Gaagige-oshkiniiigikwe *name pers* Forever Young Woman; Manidoo

gaagiigido *vai* s/he talks, s/he speaks

gaagiigidotamaw *vta* speak on behalf of h/

gaagiigidowin *ni* speech

gaagiiwozhitoo *vai* s/he wanders about

gaagiizom *vta* asks h/ for forgiveness, apologizes to h/

gaagwiinawaabaminaagozi *vai* s/he is unable to be seen, is no longer seen. Reduplication of **gwiinawaabaminaagozi**

gaagwiinawi- *pv lex* not knowing; not able. Reduplication of **gwiinawi-**

gaawiin *adv neg* no, not

gaawiin mashi *adv tmp* not yet

gaawiin wiikaa *adv tmp* never

ge- *pv tns* future tense preverb under initial change

gegapii *adv tmp* after a while, eventually, finally

geget *adv man* sure, indeed, certainly, really

gego *adv neg* don't

gego ganage *adv man* don't in any way, don't you dare

gegoo *pron indf* something, anything. *inanimate indefinite*

gemaa *adv* conj or, or maybe

gemaa gaye *adv man* or maybe

gete-anishinaabe *na* an old-time Indian, an Indian of former time

gete-gikinoo'amaadiwigamig *ni* an old school, a school of former times

geyaabi *adv tmp* still, yet

gezika *adv tmp* suddenly

gezikwendan *vti* barely remember it

gibwanaabaawe *vai* s/he drowns

gichi- *pv lex* big, great; *also* **chi-**

gichi-aya'aawi *vai* s/he is an elder

Gichi-manidoo-giizis *na* January

gidagiigin *ni* print cotton fabric

giday *na* your dog

gidimaagizi *vai* s/he is poor, is pitiful

gidisiins *nid* your navel, umbilical cord; belly button

gidoodem *nad* your clan

Giganaan *name pers* Moon; Manidoo

gigishkaw *vta* be pregnant with h/

gigitizimag *nad* your parents

gijichaagwanaan *nad* our soul (the spirit within)

gikendan *vti* know it

gikendaagwad *vii* it is known (by someone), "they" know it

gikenim *vta* know h/, know of h/

gikina'amaw *vta* forbid h/ to, warn h/ against. Reduplication of **gina'amaw**

gikinawaabam *vta* imitate h/; learn by observation of h/

gikinawaabi *vai* s/he learns from observation

gikinawaadendaagwad *vii* it is known by observation

gikinoo'amaw *vta* teach it to h/

gikinoo'amaage *vai* s/he teaches, instructs

gikinoo'amaagozi *vai* s/he goes to school

gikinoo'amaagoowizi *vai* s/he is taught

gikinoonowin *ni* year

gimishoomisinaan *na* our grandfather; powerful spirit (e.g., drum, rock, glacier)

gimoodi *vai* s/he steals

gina'amaw *vta* forbid h/ to, warn h/ against

gindidaawizi *vai* s/he is whole; **gendidawizinijn asemaan** plug tobacco

giniigaaniiminaang *nad* our future

giniigaaniiming *nad* your future

giniijaanis *nad* your child

ginoozi *vai* s/he is tall, is long

ginwaabiigizi *vai* s/he is long (as something string-like)

ginwenzh *adv tmp* for a long time

ginzhizhawizi *vai* s/he is a hard worker

gitigaazo *vai* h/ is planted

gitimi *vai* s/he is lazy, is incompetent

gitimishki *vai* s/he is habitually lazy

giwiiji-anishinaabem *nad* your fellow Anishinaabe

giwiiji-bimaadiziim *nad* your fellow human

giwiiyaw *nid* your body

gizhibaabitaw *vta* run around h/

gizhibaashkaw *vta* go around h/

gizhibaashkaamagad *vii* it goes around

gii- *pv tns* past tense

giigoonh *na* fish

gii'igoshimo *vai* s/he fasts for a vision

gii'igoshimowin *ni* fasting

giin *pron per* you (singular) *second person singular pronoun*

giinawind *pron per* we, us; *first person inclusive plural pronoun including the person or persons spoken to with the speaker*

giishkizh /giishkizhw-/ *vta* cut h/ off; cut through, cut h/

giishkizhigaazo *vai* s/he is cut off (by someone), "they" cut h/ off

giishpin *adv gram* if

giiwashkwebiishki *vai* s/he is a drunk

giiwe *vai* s/he goes home, s/he return

giiwedin *ni* north wind, north. **giiwedinong** in the north

giiwewizh *vta* take, carry h/ home

giiwose *vai* s/he hunts

giiyawen'enyiminaanig *nad* our namesakes

giizis *na* sun, moon, month

giizhaa *adv tmp* beforehand; in advance; ahead of time

giizhaajim *vta* finish telling about h/

giizhigi *vai* s/he is full grown

giizhikaandag *na* a cedar bough

giizhiikan *vii* finish, finish with it

giizhiitaa *vai* s/he finishes, gets done

gomaapii *adv deg* for some time, some distance, after awhile

goshkozi *vai* s/he wakes up, is awake

gotan *vti* be afraid of it, fear it

Gookomisakiinaan *name pers* Our Grandmother Earth
    (Wenabozho's grandmother); Manidoo

goon *na* snow

gwayak *adv man* straight, right, correct

gwaashkwani *vai* s/he jumps

gwiishkoshi *vai* s/he whistles

gwiiwizens *na* boy

gwiiwizensiwi *vai* s/he is a boy

i'iw *pron dem* that; *inanimate singular demonstrative; also* **iw**

i'iwapii *adv tmp* at that time

idash *adv conj* and; *also* **dash**

igaye *adv conj* as for, also, too, and; *also* **gaye**

igo *pc emph* [emphatic word]; *also* **-go**

ikido *vai* s/he says, s/he speaks

iko *pc asp* used to, formerly, it was the custom to; *also* **-ko**

ikwe *na* woman

ikwewi *vai* she is female

ikwezens *na* a girl

imaa *adv loc* there

inabi *vai* s/he sits a certain way, sits there

inaginde *vii* it has a certain cost, has a certain price

inagoode *vii* it hangs a certain way

ina'oonwewizi *vai* s/he is given things, is gifted a certain way

ina'oozh /ina'ooN-/ *vta* gift h/ in a certain way

inakamigizi *vai* s/he does a certain thing, has such happen to h/

inanjige *vai* s/he eats a certain way

inawem *vta* be related to h/

inawemaagan *na* a relative. **gidinawemaaganinaanig** our relatives

inawendaaso *vai* s/he is related in a certain way. **besho enawendaawasojig** close relatives

inaabadad *vii* it is useful in a certain way, is employed in a certain way

inaabaji' *vta* use h/ a certain way

inaabam *vta* see h/ a certain way as in a dream; have such a dream about h/

inaabandan *vti* see it a certain way as in a dream; have such a dream about it

inaadizi *vai* s/he has a certain character or nature, has a certain way of life

inaajimo *vai* s/he tells a certain way

inaajimotaw *vta* tell h/ of (it) a certain way

inaakonige *vai vai* s/he decides things a certain way, s/he agrees on something

inaapine *vai* s/he is sick in a certain way

inaasamabi *vai* s/he sits facing in a certain way

indedeyiban *nad-pret* my late father

inendam *vai2* s/he thinks a certain way, decides, agrees

inendamowin *ni* thoughts. **odinendamowiniwaa** their thoughts

inendan *vti* think of it a certain way

inendaagozi *vai* s/he is thought of a certain way, seem to be a certain way, have a certain destiny

inendaagwad *vii* it is thought of a certain way, seem to be a certain way; have a certain destiny

inenim *vta* think of h/ a certain way

ingiw *pron dem* those

ingo-dibik *qnt num* one night

ingoding *adv* sometime; at one time

ingodwaak *adv* one hundred

ingoji *adv deg* somewhere, anywhere, approximately, nearly

inigaachigaazo *vai* s/he is treated badly, abused, hurt (by someone), "they" treat, abuse, hurt h/

inigaa' *vta* treat h/ badly, abuse h/, hurt h/

inigaatoon *vti2* treat it badly, abuse it, hurt it

inigaawendam *vai2* s/he feels bad; depressed

inigaazi *vai* s/he is pitiful

inigokwekamig *adv qnt* abundance

inikaa *vai* s/he goes a certain way

inikaamagad *vii* s/he goes a certain way

ininamaw *vta* hand it to h/ a certain way

inini *na* a man

iniw *pron dem* that *animate obviative demonstrative;* those *inanimate plural demonstrative; also* **inow**

inow *pron dem* that *animate obviative demonstrative;* those *inanimate plural demonstrative; also* **iniw**

inwe *vai* s/he speaks a certain language

isa *pc emph* [emphatic word]; *also* **-sa**

ishke *pc disc* look! behold!

ishkose *vai* s/he is remaining; leftover

ishkose *vii* it is remaining; leftover

ishkwaa- *pv lex* after

ishkwaa-ayaa *vai* s/he has passed, is dead

ishkwaaj *adv tmp* last; finally

ishkweyaang *adv loc* behind; in the past

ishpiming *adv loc* in the sky, above

ishwaachiwag *vai* they are eight, there are eight of them

iw *pron dem* that *inanimate singular demonstrative; also* **i'iw**

iwapii *adv tmp* at that time; then

iwedi bezhig *pron dem* that other one over there

iwidi *adv loc* over there

izhaa *vai* s/he goes to a certain place

izhaamagad *vii* it goes to a certain place

izhi /iN-/ *vta* say to h/, speak so to h/

izhi- *pv lex* in a certain way, to a certain place, thus, so, there

izhi-ayaa *vai* s/he is a certain way

izhi-gwayak *adv man* straight

izhi-wiindan *vti* call it a certain way, name it a certain way

izhi-wiinjigaade *vii* it is named a certain way (by someone); "they" name it a certain way

izhi-wiinjigaazo *vai* be named a certain way (by someone); "they" name h/ a certain way

izhi-wiinzh /izhi-wiin-/ *vta* call h/ a certain way, name h/ a certain way

izhichigaadan *vti* make it a certain way

izhichigaazh /izhichigaaN-/ *vta* make h/ a certain way

izhichige *vai* s/he does things a certain way

izhi'on *ni* a sacred item used as spiritual support. **Odizhi'on** h/ sacred object

izhinan *vti* see, perceive it a certain way

izhinaw *vta* see, perceive h/ a certain way

izhinaagwad *vii* it has a certain look or appearance

izhingwashi *vai* s/he sleeps so

izhinikaazo *vai* s/he is named a certain way

izhinikaazowin *ni* a personal name

izhinizha'igaade *vii* it is sent to a certain place (by someone), "they" send it to a certain place

izhinizha'igaazo *vai* s/he is sent to a certain place (by someone), "they" send h/ to a certain place

izhise *vii* it has a certain cost, has a certain price

izhitwaa *vai* s/he has a certain custom or belief, practices a certain religion

izhiwebizi *vai* s/he behaves a certain way, s/he has certain things happen to h/, fares a certain way

izhiwinigaazo *vai* s/he is taken, carried to a certain place (by someone), "they" take, carry h/ to certain place

izhiwizh /izhiwiN-/ *vta* take, carry h/ to a certain place

jiibaakaw *vta* cook for h/

jiibaakwe *vai* s/he cooks

jiigayi'ii *adv loc* along it; by it

jiigikana *adv loc* alongside the road or trail

jiisakii *vai* s/he operates a shaking tent

madoodiswan *ni* a sweat lodge

maji-inendan *vti* think bad about it

makadeke *vai* s/he blackens h/ face with charcoal (as when fasting for a vision)

makadewaamagad *vii* it is black, is dark (in color)

makadewiingwe *vai* s/he has a dark face, a black face

mamanaajitoon *vti* treat h/ with respect, handle it carefully. Reduplication of **manaajitoon**

mamaajigaadeni *vai* s/he moves h/ legs

mamaajii *vai* s/he moves, s/he is in motion

mamaanjigozi *vai* s/he is physically disabled

mamiikwaan *vta* praise h/

mamiikwaanidizo *vat* praise h/self

mamoon *vti2* take it

manaaji' *vta* treat h/ with respect

manaajitoon *vti* treat h/ with respect, handle it carefully

manaazom *vta* speak respectfully to h/

manezi *vai+o* s/he lacks (it)

mangaanibii *vai* s/he shovels something

Manidoo *na* spirit

manidoo-aabajichigan *ni* ceremonial items

manidoo-dewe'igan *na* ceremonial drum

Manidoo-gwiiwizensag *na-pl* Little People in the Woods;
    Manidoog; *also* **Memengwesiwag**

manidoo-niimi'idiike *vai* s/he conducts a ceremonial dance

manidooke *vai* s/he conducts a ceremony

manidoominensikaan *na* an item of beadwork

manidoowaadad *vii* it has a spiritual nature

manidoowaadizi *vai* s/he has a spiritual nature

manidoowichige *vai* s/he has or participates in a ceremony

manoomin *ni* wild rice

manoominike *vai* s/he rices, goes ricing, makes rice, picks rice,
    harvests wild rice

mashi *adv tmp* yet

mashkawaadad *vii* it is strong, powerful

mashkawaadizi *vai* s/he is strong, powerful

mashkawaamagad *vii* it is powerful

mashkiki *ni* medicine

mashkimodens *ni* a small bag

mawadisidiwag *vai* they visit each other

mawadishiwe *vai* she visits people

mawi *vai* s/he cries, s/he weeps

mawidisaadan *vti* visit it

mazina'igan *ni* a book

maa *adv deg* for some time, some distance; some amount; to a
    middling degree; *also* **gomaa**

maadaginzo *vai* it is the first day (of the month)

maada'adoo *vai* s/he goes off following a trail

maada'ookii *vai+o* s/he passes (it) out

maagizhaa *adv man* maybe; I think that . . . , perhaps

maajaa *vai* s/he leaves, departs, starts off

maajaa' *vta* hold a funeral for h/

maajaa'iwe *vai* s/he holds a funeral, speaks at a funeral

maajitaa *vai* s/he starts an activity

maajii- *pv lex* start; begin; start off

maajiidoon *vti2* carry, take it away

maajiigin *vii* it starts growing, grows up

maajiikamigaa *vii* it is the future

maakishkoozo *vai* s/he is shot and wounded

maamakaadendam *vai2* s/he is amazed, is baffled

maamandoogwaason *ni* a hand-sewn quilt

maamawinikeniwag *vai* they put their hands together

maamiigiwe *vai* s/he gives something, gives things away

maamiijin *vti3* keep eating it. Reduplication of **miijin**

maazhi-doodaw *vta* treat h/ badly

maazhi-izhiwebizi *vai* s/he behaves badly

maazhichige *vai* s/he does wrong, does bad things

maazhise *vai* s/he has something bad happen to h/

megwaa *adv tmp* while; during; right now

megwe- *pv lex* among, in the midst of. **megwe-biboon** during the
winter, in the midst of winter

memengwesiwag *na-pl* Little People in the Woods; Manidoog;
also **Manidoo-gwiiwizensag**

memwech *adv man* just that, exactly, it is so. **gaawiin memwech**
it is not necessary

meshkwadoonigan *na* money

mewinzha *adv tmp* a long time ago, long ago

michi- *pv* by hand; without anything special

michi-giizhitoon *vti* create it

midewi *vai* s/he is a Mide, is a member of the Midewiwin

midewi'iwe *vai* s/he conducts a Midewiwin ceremony for people

migwanaadizi *vai* s/he is unsettled within

mikan *vti* find it

mikaw *vta* find h/

mikwam *na* ice

mikwendan *vti* remember it, recollect it, come to think of it

mikwenim *vta* remember h/, recollect h/, come to think of h/

minawaanigwendam *vai2* s/he feels happy, feels glad

mindido *vai* s/he is big

mindimooyenh *na* old lady, old woman

minik *adv qnt* a certain amount, a certain number, so much, so many

minikwe *vai+o* s/he drinks (it)

minikwewin *ni* alcohol, drink

Minisinaakwaang *name place* East Lake

minjimenim *vta* keep h/ in h/ mind, remember h/

minjiminan *vti* hold on to it

mino-ayaawin *ni* good health

mino-doodaw *vta* treat h/ well

mino-mamaajiiwin *ni* good movement

minochige *vai* s/he does well, does a good thing

minokaw- *vta* [inverse] it (something consumed) agrees with h/, does h/ good

minwaabadad *vii* it is useful, is of good use

minwendam *vai2* s/he is happy, is joyous, is glad, has a good time

minwendan *vti* like it

minwii *vai* s/he moves easily, works without distraction, is efficient

misawaa *adv gram* no matter what; even though, even if, despite

misawaabam *vta* look with desire at h/, want to have h/

misawendan *vti* desire, want it

Misi-zaaga'igan *name place* Mille Lacs Reservation, Minnesota

miskozi *vai* s/he is red

miskwegad *vii* it is red (as something sheet-like)

miskwi *ni* blood

mitadaawangaa *vii* it is bare ground

mitig *na* a tree

mitigwaab *na* a bow

mii *adv pred* it is thus that, it is that

mii dash *adv conj* and then

miigaadiwag /miigaadi-/ *vai* they fight each other. **endazhi-miigaading** the war

miigiwe *vai* s/he gives something, gives things away

miigwan *na* a feather

miigwechiwendam *vai2* s/he is thankful, is grateful

miigwechiwi' *vta* thank h/

miigwechiwitaagozi *vai* s/he gives thanks

miijin *vti3* eat it

miikana *ni* a road, a trail, a path

miikanens *ni* path, road

miikinzom *vta* provoke, tease, harass h/ (by voice)

miinawaa *adv conj* again, and, also; *also* **naa**

miinigoowizi *vai* s/he is given (in a spiritual way)

miizh *vta* give (it) h/

moonendan *vti* realize, sense it

moonenim *vta* sense h/

moonike *vai* s/he digs a hole or burrow

mooshkina' *vta* fill h/ (with solids)

moozhag *adv tmp* often, constantly, several times

na *pc disc* [yes-no question word]. *also* **ina**

Nabaanaabe *na* Mermaid; a Manidoo

nagamotaw *vta* sing to h/

nagazh /nagaN/ *vta* leave h/ behind; abandon h/

nagishkaw *vta* meet h/ (while going somewhere)

na'aanganikwe *na* a daughter-in-law

na'inigaazo *vai* s/he is put away (by someone); "they" put h/ away; s/he is buried

nakodan *vti* answer it

nakwetaw *vta* answer h/

namanj *adv dub* I don't know how, I wonder how; *also* **amanj**

namebin *na* sucker (fish)

nanagin *vta* hold h/ back; prevent h/ (from doing something)

nanaa'inigaazo *vai* s/he is put away (by someone); "they" put h/ away; s/he is buried. Reduplication of **na'inigaazo**

nanaamadabi *vai* s/he sits, sits down. Reduplication of
   namadabi
nanaandawi' *vta* heal, h/doctor
nanaandawi'iwe *vai* s/he heals, doctors people
nanaandom *vta* ask for, call, summon h/. Reduplication of
   nandom
nanaandonge *vai* s/he requests things. Reduplication
   of **nandonge**
nanaapaadakizine *vai* s/he puts a shoes on the wrong feet
nandawaabandan *vti* look for, search for it
nandobijige *vai* s/he is searching, feeling for thing with hands
nandodamaage *vai* s/he asks people, begs people for things
nandom *vta* ask h/ for, call, summon h/
nandwewem *vta* go and ask for h/
nandwewendan *vti* go and ask for it
naniibikim *vta* scold h/
naniizaanendan *vti* think it dangerous
naniizaanendaagwad *vii* it is considered dangerous
naniizaanenim *vta* think h/ dangerous
napaazi-zagaakwa'an *vti* fasten, pin, button it the wrong way
nawaj *adv deg* more
Nazhike'awaasong *pers name* The Evening Star—The One That
   Shines Alone; Manidoo
Nazhikewigaabawiikwe *name pers* Sophia Churchill-Benjamin
naa *adv conj* again, and, also; *also* **miinawaa**
naa *pc emph* [emphatic word] well
naabibiitaw *vta* take h/ place, sit as a representative of h/, par-
   take in a ceremony in h/ seat
naabishkaage *vai* s/he accepts or takes something for someone,
   partakes in an offering on someone else's behalf
naadamaw *vta* help h/
naadamaage *vai* s/he helps people
naadamaagoowizi *vai* s/he is helped (in a spiritual way)
naanaagadawendamowin *ni* thoughts

naanaagandawendam *vai2* s/he considers, notices, thinks, reflects, realizes

naaning *adv* five times

naanoopinadoon *vti2* follow it, go after it (something moving). Reduplication of **noopinadoon**

naawayi'ii *adv tmp* in the middle

naazikan *vti* go to it, approach it

naazikaw *vta* go to, approach h/

naazikaage *vai* s/he goes to people, approaches people

nebowa *adv qnt* many, much; a lot

Nechii'awaasong *name pers* Mary Churchill-Benjamin

Neyaashiing *name place* Vinland, Minnesota

ni- *pv lex* going away, going along, in progress, on the way, coming up in time; *also* **ani**

nibaa *vai* s/he sleeps, is asleep

nibaadizi *vai* s/he is a greedy eater, is gluttonous

nibi *ni* water

nibiikaa *vii* there is (a lot of) water

nichiiwad *vii* there is a severe storm

nichiiwenimo *vai* s/he is a bully, acts tough, is aggressive

nigitiziimag *nad* my parents

nigozis *nad* my son

nimaamaayiban *nad-pret* my late mother

nindaanis *nad* my daughter

ningaabii'an *ni* west. **ningaabii'anong** in the west

niniigaaniiming *nad* my future

niniijaanisens *nad* my infant

ninjiid *nid* my anus

ninoshenh *nad* my aunt (mother's sister)

nisidawinaagwad *vii* it is known, recognized, identifies (by sight)

nisidizo *vai* s/he kills h/ self, commits suicide

nising *adv tmp* three times

niso-dibik *qnt num* three nights

nishi /niS-/ *vta* kill h/

nishwanaadizi *vai* s/he is deviating from normal behavior

nishwanaaji-ikido *vai* s/he says things that do not make sense

nishwanaaji' *vta* waste, spoil, destroy h/

nishwanaajitoon *vti2* waste, spoil, destroy it

nishwanaajiwebinige *vai* s/he makes a mess of things, does not do things correctly

nitam *adv loc* first

nitaa- *pv lex* know how to do something; being good at; being skilled at; frequently do

nitaage *vai* s/he kills game, kills people, murders

nitaawichige *vai* s/he is skilled at something, knows how to make things

nitaawigi' *vta* grow h/, raise h/

nitoon *vti2* kill it

niwiij'aya'aa *na* my sibling (male or female)

niwiiji-anishinaabe *nad* my fellow Anishinaabe

nizigosiban *nad-pret* my late aunt (cross-aunt: father's sister)

nizhishenyiban *nad-pret* my late uncle (cross-uncle: mother's brother)

niibawi *vai* s/he stands

niibawitaw *vta* stand up for h/

niibaa-dibik *adv tmp* late at night

niibidebi' *vta* seat h/ side by side in a row

niibinaakwaanininj *ni* a finger

niigaan *adv loc* ahead, leading, at the front; in the future

Niigaani-manidoo *name pers* head Manidoo; Manidoo

niigaanii *vai* s/he goes ahead, leads

niimi *vai* s/he dances

niimi'idiwag /niimi'idi-/ *vai* they dance

niimi'idiike *vai* s/he conducts a ceremonial dance

niimi'iwewinini *na* a singer

niin *pron per* I, me *first person singular pronoun*

niiskaadad *vii* it is bad weather

niishitana *adv num* twenty

niishtana-biboonagizi *vai* s/he is twenty years old

niitaawis *nad* my close male relative (male speaking)

niiwaak *qnt num* four hundred

niiwing *adv tmp* four times

niiwiwag *vai* they are four, there are four of them

niiwo-dibik *qnt num* four nights

niiwo-giiziswagizi *vai* s/he is four months old

niiwo-giizhigad *vii* it is the fourth day

niiyawen'enh *nad* my namesake

niiyo-dibik *qnt num* four nights

niizh *qnt num* two

niizhing *adv tmp* two times, twice

niizho-dibik *qnt num* two nights

niizhwaasimidana *qnt num* seventy

noobaajigaade *vii* it is suckled on (by someone), "they" suckle on it

noodendam *vai2* s/he flirts

noogitaa *vai* s/he stops an activity, stops working

noomaya *adv tmp* recently; a while ago; a little while ago

noondan *vti* hear it

noonde-nibaa *vai* s/he falls asleep (before the usual time)

noongom *adv tmp* now, nowadays, today

o- *pv dir* going to somewhere to do something

Obizaan *pers name* Lee Staples

odamino *vai* s/he plays

odaminwaagaansi-zhiishiigwan *ni* a small toy rattle (in contrast to a ceremonial rattle)

odaabaan *na* a car

odaapinan *vti* accept it, take

odedeyan *nad* h/ father

odedeyi *vai+o* s/he has a father

ode' *nid* h/ heart
odengwayaang *nid* on h/ face
odisiins *nid* h/ navel, belly button, umbilical cord
odish /odiS-/ *vta* come upon h/, visit h/, meet up with h/
oditan *vti* come up to, reach it
odiyaang *nid* on h/ rear end, butt
odizhi'on *nid* h/ sacred object
ogijayi'ii *adv loc* on top of it
Ogimaawab *name pers* John Benjamin
ogitiziiman *nad* h/ parents
ogitiziimiwaabanen *nad-pret* their late parent/parents
ogitiziimiwaan *nad* their parents
ogoodaasiwaan *nid* their dresses
ogookomisan *nad* h/ grandmother/grandmothers
o'ow *pron dem* this. *inanimate singular demonstrative*
ojaanimizi *vai* s/he is busy
ojibwemo *vai* s/he speaks Ojibwe
ojibwemotaw *vta* speak Ojibwe to h/
Ojibwemowin *ni* the Ojibwe language
ojichaagoshin *vai* s/he (someone's spirit) leaves an impression
ojichaagwan *nad* h/ soul (h/ spirit within)
ojiibik *ni* a root
ojiid *nid* h/ anus
ojiim *vta* kiss h/
okaakigan *nid* h/ chest
okosijige *vai* s/he makes a bundle; s/he piles, stacks things
okwi'idiwag /okwi'idi-/ *vai* they get together
omakakii *na* a frog
omaa *adv loc* here
omaamaayan *nad* h/ mother
omaamaayi *vai+o* s//he has a mother
ombin *vta* lift, raise it
ombiigwewetoo *vai* s/he is loud

omigii *vai* s/he has a sore or sores, has a scab or scabs

Omigiinaans *name pers* a character in a winter legend, Scabby Boy

omigiiwin *ni* a scab (referring to dried-up umbilical cord)

omoodens *ni* a small bottle

onabi' *vta* seat h/, appoint h/

onagaakizid *nid* h/ sole

onaabam *vta* select h/

onaabeman *nad* her husband

onaagan *ni* dish, plate

onaagaans *ni* cup

onaajiwan *vii* it is beautiful

onda'ibii *vai* s/he gets, draws water from a certain place

ondanjige *vai* s/he eats from there, gets h/ food from there

ondaadizi *vai* s/he is born, s/he comes from a certain place

ondinan *vti* get it from a certain place, obtain it from a certain place

ondinigaade *vii* it is obtained from a certain place (by someone); "they" get, obtain it from a certain place

ondinige *vai* s/he gets things from a certain place, obtains something from a certain place

ongow *pron dem* these (animate plural)

oninj *nid* h/ hand

oninjiinsiwaan *nid* their little hands

oniigaaniiming *nid* h/ future

oniigaaniimiwaang *nad* their future

oniijaanisan *nad* h/ child/children

oniijaanisensan *nad* h/ infant/infants

oniijaanisensiwaan *nad* their infant/infants

oniijaanisi *vai* s/he has a child or children, has a young one or young. **weniijaanisijig** parents

oniijaanisiwaan *nad* their child/children

onji *adv conj* because of, reason for

onji- *pv* from a certain place, for a certain reason; because

onjikaa *vai* s/he comes from a certain place

onjikaamagad *vii* it comes from a certain place

onjitaw *vta* listens to h/ from a certain place

onjii *vai* s/he comes from a certain place

onzaabam *vta* watches h/ from a certain place

onzaam *adv qnt* too, too much, excessively, extremely; because

onzaamichige *vai* s/he does things to an excessive degree, an unwanted degree

onzaamidoon *vai* s/he talks too much

opimekana *adv loc* along the side of the road or trail

opwaagan *na* a ceremonial pipe

oshkaabewis *na* helper (in a ceremony); ceremonial drum position

oshki- *pv lex* new, young, fresh, for the first time

oshki-bimaadizi *vai* s/he is young, is an adolescent

oshki-bimaadiziim *na* someone young, adolescent.
    gidooshki-bimaadiziiminaanig our young people

Oshki-daagishkang i'iw aki *ni-v* welcoming ceremony for a newborn done four days after birth

oshki-inini *na* young man, an adolescent boy

oshki-ininiwi *vai* he is a young man, an adolescent boy

oshkiniigikwe *na* a young woman, an adolescent girl

oshkiinzhig *nid* h/ eye

oshtigwaan *nid* h/ head

ow *pron dem* this; also **o'ow**

owapii *adv tmp* at this time, then

owiiji-anishinaabemiwaan *nad* their fellow Indian/Indians, their Anishinaabe/Anishinaabeg

owiiji-bimaadiziiman *nad* h/ fellow human being/human beings

owiinizisan *nid* h/ hair

owiiyaw *nid* h/ body

owiiyawen'enyimiwaan *nad* their namesake or namesakes

ozidensan *nid* h/ little feet

ozhibii'an *vti* write it, write it down

ozhibii'igaade *vii* it is written (by someone), "they" write it; it is written down (by someone), "they" write it down

ozhichigaade *vii* it is made, built, formed (by someone), "they" make, build, form it

ozhige *vai* s/he builds a dwelling (lodge, house), makes camp

ozhi' *vta* make, build, form h/

ozhitamaw *vta* make, build, form (it) for h/

ozhitoon *vti2* make it, build it, create it

ozhiitaa *vai* s/he gets ready, prepares

wa! *pc disc* [exclamation of agreeable surprise] awesome!, great!, excellent!

wadiswan *ni* a nest

wanendan *vti* forget, ignore it

wanenim *vta* forget, ignore h/

wani' *vta* lose, miss h/

waniba' *vta* [inverse] it eludes h/

wanichige *vai* s/he makes a mistake, makes things wrong

wanishin *vai* s/he is lost, gets lost

wanishkwe' *vta* disturb, distract, interrupt h/

wanishkwem *vta* disturb, distract, interrupt h/ (by speech)

wanitaaso *vai* s/he loses someone

wanitoon *vti2* lose, miss it

wapii *adv tmp* at that time

wawaaj *adv man* and even

wawenabi *vai* s/he is sitting down, stays seated

wawenabi' *vta* seat h/

wawiyazh *adv man* funny; comical

wawiinge- *pv lex* properly; carefully; completely; well; biological. **niwawiinge-maamaayiban** my biological mother [*nad-pret*]

wawiingezi *vai* s/he is skillful, does a good job, does something well

wayeshkad *adv tmp* at first; in the beginning

wayezhim *vta* cheat h/

waa- *pv tns* [future tense prefix under initial change]

waabam *vta* see h/

waabanda' *vta* show (it) to h/

waabanda'igoowizi *vai* s/he is shown

waabanda'iwe *vai* s/he shows something to people

waabandan *vti* see it

waabanjigaade *vii* it is seen (by someone), "they" see it

waabanjigaazo *vai* s/he is seen (by someone), "they" see it

waabi *vai* s/he has vision

waabishkiiwe *vai* s/he is a white person

waabooyaan *ni* blanket

waabooz *na* a rabbit

waakaabiitaw *vta* sit around h/

waakaa'igaans *ni* a bathroom, restroom

waanaji' *vta* have a lot of h/

waasa *adv loc* far, far away, distant

waawan *ni* an egg

waawaabanjigaazo *vai* s/he is seen (by someone), "they" see it. Reduplication of **waabanjigaazo**

waawaashkeshi *na* a deer

waawaashkeshiwi-wiiyaas *ni* deer meat, venison

waawiindamaw *vta* tell h/ about (it), explain (it) to h/, promise (it) to him

waawiindaawaso *vai* s/he names a child, gives names, has a naming ceremony. Reduplication of **wiindaawaso**

waazakonenjiganaaboo *ni* gasoline

Wenabozho *name pers* the Manidoo who once lived among us as a man

wenda- *pv lex* really; completely; just so; especially

wenipanizi *vai* s/he does something easily

wenjida *adv man* especially, particularly, above all

wewebanaabii *vai* s/he fishes with a hook and line

weweni *adv man* in a good way, properly, correctly, carefully, safely

wewiib *adv man* hurry, in a hurry, quickly

wii- *pv tns* is going to, will, want to

wiidookaw *vta* help h/

wiidoopam *vta* eat with h/, share food with h/

wiigiwaam *ni* wigwam

wiigwaas-asemaa-onaagan *ni* a birch bark tobacco dish

wiij'ayaaw *vta* be with h/, live or stay with h/

wiiji' *vta* play with h/

wiiji'aagan *na* playmate

wiiji'iwe *vai* s/he goes with, accompanies people

wiijiwaagan *na* a partner, a companion

wiijiiw *vta* go with h/, accompany h/

wiikaa *adv tmp* late; ever; seldom

wiikwajitoon *vti2* try to do it, make an effort to do it

wiin *pron per* he, she; her, him; *third person singular pronoun*

wiinawaa *pron per* they, them; *third person plural personal pronoun*

wiindamaw *vta* tell h/ about (it)

wiindamaage *vai* s/he tells about (it) to people, explains (it) to people

wiindamaagoowizi *vai* s/he is told

wiindan *vti* name it, mention the name of it

wiindaawaso *vai* s/he names a child, gives names, has a naming ceremony

wiinitam *pron per* his turn, her turn, him next

wiipem *vta* sleep with h/

wiisagishin *vai* s/he gets hurt (on something), gets hurt falling

wiisini *vai* s/he eats

wiisiniwin *ni* food

wiishkoba'igaade *vii* it is sweetened (by someone), "they" sweeten it

wiiyawen'enyan *nad* h/ namesake (reciprocal relationship between name-giving sponsor and child)

wiiyawen'enyi *vai* h/ has a namesake or namesakes

wiiyawen'enyikaw *vta* give h/ an Anishinaabe name; give him namesakes

wiiyawen'enyikaage *vai* s/he gives people an Anishinaabe name

wiiyaas *ni* meat; a piece of meat

zagaswaa *vai* s/he smokes (tobacco)

zagaswe'idiwag /zagaswe'idi-/ *vai* they have a feast or ceremony

zakab *adv man* at peace, quiet

zanagad *vii* it is difficult, it is hard to manage

zazaagizi *vai* s/he is stingy

zazegaatoon *vti2* dress it up

zaziikizi *vai* s/he is the eldest

zaaga'am *vai2* s/he goes to the toilet

zaaga'igan *ni* lake

zaagewe *vai* s/he comes suddenly into view (as from around the corner)

zegi' *vta* scare, frighten h/

zegingwashi *vai* s/he has a nightmare

zenibaanh *na* ribbon

zinigobidoon *vti2* rub, massage it with something

ziibi *ni* river

ziinzibaakwadoons *ni* candy

ziinzibaakwadwaapine *vai* s/he has diabetes

zhakamoozh /zhakamooN-/ *vta* spoon-feed h/

zhawendaagozi *vai* s/he is shown compassion, is pitied (by someone), "they" show compassion to, pity h/

zhawendaagoziwin *ni* compassion

zhawenim *vta* have compassion for h/, pity h/

zhazhiibitam *vai2* s/he is stubborn, is disobedient

zhaaganaashiimo *vai* s/he speaks English

zhaashaagwam *vta* chew on h/

zhiginidizo *vai* s/he urinates on h/ self

zhimaaganishiiwi *vai* s/he is a soldier
zhingishin *vai* s/he is lying down
zhingwaak *na* a pine
zhiigwaakonan *vti* exclude it, rule it out
zhiigwaakozh /zhiigwaakoN-/ *vta* exclude h/, rule h/ out
zhiingitaw *vta* dislike, hate listening to or hearing h/
zhooniiyaans *na* money